PRAISE FOR
SURF THE~~RAPY~~

~~eee~~

"Cash expertly balances storytelling with scientific rigor, making complex concepts accessible to both the seasoned surf therapy practitioner and the armchair adventurer. This book is not just a literary journey—it's an invitation to ride the waves within and discover the transformative power that awaits us in the sea's embrace."

—KRIS PRIMACIO, CEO of the International
Surf Therapy Organization (ISTO)

"*Surf Therapy* is the expression of energy as a wave meets the shore. Nothing but applause for Lambert's efforts in so eloquently telling our story and sharing it with the world."

—DR. CARLY M ROGERS, OTD, OTR/L, creator of
Ocean Therapy & Founding Director of Programs
for the Jimmy Miller Memorial Foundation

"Cash blends beautiful storytelling, cutting edge science, and emotive personal testimony to explore the life changing potential of the emerging surf therapy sector."

—DR. JAMIE MARSHALL, Research Fellow at
Edinburgh Napier University.

"Everything in this book flows—from the narrative voice to the voices of the surfing storytellers, from oceans to health clinics, from bodies to souls—*Surf Therapy* is another healing gift from author Cash Lambert."

—DAVID ATHEY, Professor of English, Palm Beach Atlantic
University & author of *Above the Harbor*

"In *Surf Therapy*, Cash Lambert does an expert job of blending emotional testimonials and definitive data to reveal exactly that. This book digs deep into surf therapy. It's an excellent read for anyone seeking hope, healing, and an adrenaline rush."

—JAMIE BRISICK, author of
Birth of the Endless Summer: A Surf Odyssey

"Deconstructing the modern theories and practices of surf therapy and the multitude of ways it's being applied today, for anyone looking to move forward in life, find a little peace and ride a few waves in the process, it's a must-read."

—JAKE HOWARD, writer for
Sports Illustrated and *Surfer Magazine*

"Here in these pages, [Cash] visits with surf therapy practitioners, participants and volunteers, and shines compelling light on the essential work being done in and around the water to bring about meaningful change in the lives of families on the spectrum and others."

—DANIEL PAISNER, co-author of
Scratching the Horizon: A Surfing Life

"From tortured vets suffering PTSD to addicts in recovery to homeless children searching for direction, *Surf Therapy* is the fascinating story of just how cathartic the act of riding waves was than we'd ever imagined."

—BEAU FLEMISTER, author of *In the Seat of a Stranger's Car*

"*Surf Therapy* is a masterful exploration of the benefits, practices, and potential of surfing to change lives for the better."

—BRAD HOOK, partner at the Resilience Institute
and founder of *Surfd*

surf
therapy

surf therapy

THE EVIDENCE-BASED SCIENCE FOR PHYSICAL, MENTAL & EMOTIONAL WELL-BEING

Cash Lambert

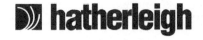

SURF THERAPY

Library of Congress Cataloging-in-Publication Data is available.
ISBN: 978-1-57826-994-5

Cover and Interior Design by Carolyn Kasper

Printed in the United States
10 9 8 7 6 5 4 3 2 1

*To the surf therapy community—past,
present, and future—may this book
help those in need benefit
from the ocean's healing waves now and forevermore.*

CONTENTS

Introduction

ℓℓℓ

The 21st century was envisioned as an unprecedented time of opportunity and advancement, both of which would lead to a healthier human body. Less pain, less suffering, less disease; and thus, more universal happiness.

What a stark contrast it is to see that imaginary future against the realities of our present 21st century lives.

We have such high levels of mental illness—PTSD, anxiety, depression and more—that it is widely considered a mental health crisis;[1] more than half of all women will be exposed to at least one traumatic event in their lifetime;[2] and rates of autism are at their highest in recorded history.[3] Military service men and women have returned home from active duty with increased rates of PTSD, alarming rates of suicide and other injuries. Because of this, the Veteran Affairs and Centers for Disease Control and Prevention have declared a National Health Crisis in the United States.

Disabilities have increased, compared to the previous century.[4] The rate of refugees—due to persecution, violence, conflict, among others—has steadily climbed to an all-time high in this century,[5] which can lead to increased risk for trauma and other mental illnesses.

Traditional western medicine has aimed to treat all of this. But, given the sustained and continued rise of mental illness, trauma, and addiction—along with unwanted side effects from some of these traditional therapies—many have sought help through alternative, nature-based interventions.

One of those methods is surf therapy.

Surfing? You mean, the act of riding a surfboard is actually therapy?

I had the same raised-eyebrow reaction when I first heard about it, too. Yes, when the act of surfing is combined with therapeutic activities, it's proven to be therapeutic. Who knew?

The International Surf Therapy Organization defines surf therapy as, "The use of surfing as a vehicle for delivering intentional, inclusive, population-specific, and evidenced-based therapeutic structures to promote psychological, physical, and psychosocial well-being."[6]

Today, it's used around the world to combat mental illness, trauma, drug abuse, and much more—with surprising, evidence-based results.

And it's something that I've witnessed firsthand.

ecec

Surfing… a form of therapy?

It sounded odd.

As an avid surfer, I had never thought of it being therapeutic. I surfed hurricane swells in Florida, crowded peaks in Southern California, and some of the biggest waves of my life on Oahu's fabled North Shore. In the water, I felt adrenaline fueling a flow state as I paddled and dropped into waves. And after I paddled in towards shore and exited the water, I felt calmer and more relaxed. So, when I heard about surf therapy in 2010, I was curious to learn more.

I traveled to Jacksonville Beach, Florida, and from 8am-5pm on a Saturday, watched as children with autism rode waves to shore with the help of volunteers. As a freshman journalism major at Palm Beach Atlantic University, I had brought a camera and a voice recorder. If there was much to the story, I figured I would write something for the school newspaper. If not, I'd just volunteer and enjoy the day.

I quickly found out that there was much more than a story—lives were being changed, and it was happening in real time.

After watching a few rounds of children surfing, I met a boy named Spenser, and as soon as I heard his story, I knew I had to write about it.

> *"Around several parts of Florida, Spenser "Big Wave" Schwartz is a well-known surfer. The 8-year-old travels with his family to surfing events, is characterized by his charisma and humor, and is even sponsored by Boca Java Coffee, with his picture imprinted on many bags. But Schwartz is not the average surfer, and he does not attend average surf events. He has been diagnosed with autism."[7]*

I didn't realize the effects surfing had on Spenser until I spoke with his mother for the article.

> *"When he surfs, we don't see the anxiety in him,' she said. 'Instead, we see huge glow in his face.' … '[The event] changed my life, and every volunteer that I talk to,' she said. 'If you attend one of these events, it'll change you and you'll be hooked."[8]*

After she told me this, I walked around the beach talking to volunteers, families, and participants, and they echoed everything his mother had said—they were hooked. Surf therapy was indeed helping those on the autism spectrum.

But it still didn't make sense to me. I was hearing testimonials that riding a wave was not only therapeutic, but life changing, and I couldn't help but wonder how.

I had no idea that, standing on Jacksonville Beach in 2010, that question—how is surfing therapeutic?—would lead to years of research, two books, friendships born from surfing, and, most of all, a shocking, evidence-based answer.

eee

After my first surf therapy experience, I attended more surf therapy events with Surfers for Autism, who put on the event in Jacksonville Beach, and continued to do so up and down Florida's coast.

At each event, I would volunteer and write an article. These articles followed a similar template: starting by setting the scene on the beach: a participant riding waves of healing. Next, talking with a parent, likely their mother, telling me how surfing was life changing. After that, I would include statistics about the ever-growing prevalence of autism. Finally, I would end the article with some quotes from volunteers about how giving was therapeutic for them as well.

I walked away from each event with more words than could be published. After this template repeated for a few years, it was clear that if I wanted to tell the true surf therapy story I was witnessing at events, I would have to venture outside of newspapers and magazines where word counts were limited—and into a book.

So, a few weeks before walking across the stage with my hard-earned degree in journalism, I committed to spending a year entrenched with the surf therapy organization in order to answer my burning question: how was surfing therapeutic for children and young adults with autism?

What followed was years of travel up and down Florida's coast; sitting in family living rooms and hearing heartbreaking stories of diagnosis while flipping through a family photo album; attending therapy with participants; sitting in hotel hallways with parents who had put their children to sleep and enjoying their hilarious stories.

There was "Nate the Great," diagnosed with nonverbal autism. I watched how surfing helped calm his shaky nerves on the event day—and for weeks after. I also was there to witness him stand on a surfboard for the first time while his mother tearfully watched.

There was Abigail, diagnosed with infantile autism, who found happiness and friends within the surf therapy community.

There was Damian, diagnosed on the high functioning end of the spectrum, who found a passion in surfing—and even began competing with the Special Olympics surf team.

There were Ethan and Evan, twin boys on the spectrum, who gained a confidence boost through surfing—and a community they would find identity in.

There was Christopher, diagnosed with cerebral palsy and nonverbal autism, who found the thrill and adrenaline of surfing therapeutic.

I compiled all of this, and what I experienced into *Waves of Healing: How Surfing Changes the Lives of Children with Autism,* published by Hatherleigh Press in partnership with Penguin Random House.

After the book's release in 2019, I received a phone call from Kris Primacio, who introduced herself as the CEO of the International Surf Therapy Organization (ISTO). I had never heard of it before and had no idea that there were surf therapy organizations around the world. She invited me to speak at the 2019 ISTO Surf Therapy Symposium in Los Angeles, and a few months later at the conference, I sat on stage and told the emotional stories of what I witnessed to an audience of a few hundred—stories about children with autism who were labeled nonverbal speaking my name; stories of children with autism breaking barriers out of the water because they learned how to do so in the water; stories of healing.

I was used to attending surf therapy events and writing about it, so I decided to write an event recap for the surf media company, Surfline. To do so, I stuck around the event and listened to the other guest speakers. And what I heard shocked me.

They told stories of how surfing was therapeutic for veterans with PTSD, inner city children in America, refugees, children in townships in South Africa; those struggling with mental illness; women healing from trauma and more populations. In addition, there was growing evidence of surf therapy in academia.

I couldn't ask enough questions fast enough.

Dane Gudauskas, a pro surfer, recognizable by incredible front and backside skill on a wave, blonde hair, and a bright smile, had this to say about the conference:

> *"As a surfer, you inherently feel that connection and natural healing essence of surfing... but to see it with so many people in the community from all aspects of people dealing with trauma... it's amazing to hear it all come together and bridge that. There's so many heroes in that room that are phenomenal. Think about all the kind of evolution that is going to come out of something like this."[9]*

Gudauskas was right—a meeting of this many minds, who he called "heroes," was going to be kerosene on the flame that was surf therapy. Aaron Chang, a renowned photographer based in California, agreed.

> *"I think this can permeate through the medical world, throughout industries, and this can be the start of a whole new awareness ... Something that all of us who surf understand—that maybe don't articulate well—is that it feels good to be in the water. We can't explain it. We feel better every time we go in the water. I think these people [at the conference] have the academic training and skill sets to give that feeling a definition and deploy it where it can help a lot of people."[10]*

Because of my research, I knew surfing was therapeutic for autism. But I had no idea it was therapeutic for so many wide-ranging populations. On top of that, surf therapy was picking up steam. There was palpable momentum in the air.

The same question that was the genesis of *Waves of Healing* then entered my mind: How is it therapeutic for these populations?

How is surfing therapeutic for children in townships, for police officers in the line of duty, those struggling with addictions, veterans running from the memories of war, children in low-income housing areas in America, women healing from trauma?

Most importantly, is there any evidence to back it all up?

That's how the first hints of this book started.

Writing this book, I threw myself into the deep end—a bottomless pool of history, testimonials, and groundbreaking scientific studies. Collecting everything I've learned within its pages has been an absolute joy, one I'm delighted to share with you now.

Here's a glimpse into what the future holds:

In **Chapter 1: The Origins of Surf Therapy,** you will read about the beginnings of surfing as therapy, starting with the hints left behind by Native Hawaiians about their own practices. You'll also learn about the first recorded instance we have of surf therapy being used per ISTO's definition in the 21st century (a story that will surely melt your heart).

In **Chapter 2: War, PTSD & Surf Therapy for Military Service Members,** you'll read about how surfing is currently being used to combat the physical and mental scars from war on both coasts in the United States—with lifesaving results. You'll also meet three incredible women who pioneered groundbreaking surf therapy research for this population by providing some of the sector's initial research.

In **Chapter 3: Inner Cities, Townships & Radiation Zones: Surf Therapy for At-Risk Youth,** you'll experience the powerful stories of how surfing is being used to help children and young adults in low-income housing in the United States, townships in South Africa, and near the radiation zone of Chernobyl. What's more, you'll discover the incredible data that shows how toxic societal stress can be for these individuals—and how surfing can help it improve.

In **Chapter 4: Trauma Therapy, Vitamin Sea & Surf Therapy for Women Healing From Trauma,** you'll read about how one surf therapy organization has been utilizing surfing to help women suffering from a wide range of ailments and circumstances, including sex trafficking, abuse, addiction, and more. Thanks to this organization's commitment to training others in the surf therapy sector, many other organizations have come to fruition—including one that helps female Syrian refugees heal from the trauma they've endured using surfboards and saltwater.

In **Chapter 5: Incarceration, Drug Abuse & How to Live for More,** you'll read about how one man replaced his dopamine-fueled drug addiction with the dopamine-fueled nature of surfing, which helped him escape a lifestyle of incarceration—and saved his life. You'll also share in my experiences from the ISTO Surf Therapy Symposium in 2019, where I heard tear-jerking stories about an organization that takes young adults from New Zealand, trapped in a cycle of incarceration and drug addiction surfing, and helps them work towards a healthier life.

In **Chapter 6: Sirens, PTSD & Surf Therapy for Police Officers,** you'll read about how surfing (which has a historical reputation for being anti-establishment, let's be honest) is helping police officers struggling with on-the-job PTSD. You'll also find out how they were able to convince the police force in the country to have their surf therapy program tax-funded. (Here's a hint, though: irrefutable, evidence-based data is involved).

In **Chapter 7: The Spectrum, A Breath of Life & How Surfing Helps Those With Disabilities,** you'll learn about the original surf camp for autism which united children on the autism spectrum with pro surfers for an unforgettable experience. You'll also read the incredible story of two brothers, both passionate surfers, who learned the fascinating science behind how surfing—and breathing in salt air—is therapeutic for those with cystic fibrosis. Those two brothers went on to start an organization that became a movement, which has helped thousands of participants.

In **Chapter 8: Spinal Cord Injuries, Adaptive Surfboards & Surf Therapy for Physical Injuries,** you'll read the inspirational tale of how Jesse Billauer turned tragedy into triumph. You'll also learn the incredible story behind today's modern adaptive surf equipment which has paved the way for those with spinal cord injuries to surf safely.

With mental illness on the rise in both England and Australia, several practitioners have taken it upon themselves to break out of the traditional clinical setting of four walls and instead conduct therapy on the beach—and they've seen powerful, life-saving results. You'll read about the first instance of surfing being prescribed by doctors—in **Chapter 9: Surf Therapy Prescribed, Mental Health by Stealth & Surf Therapy for Mental Health.**

In **Chapter 10: Wave Pools, Inland Surfing & The Future of Surf Therapy,** you'll read about one person's vision for wave pools as mental health centers of the future. After all, surf therapy would seem to be available only to those who live or travel to the coast, an exclusive group of people. But with the current wave pool arms race—and the creation of wave pools inland—surf therapy is being offered inland populations who otherwise wouldn't have the chance to visit the coast.

The creation of this book was quite a time-consuming undertaking, but sharing the fruits of those labors with you is what makes it all worth it. As I spoke to the pioneers, living legends, and passionate practitioners of the surf therapy industry, I wondered if they, too, might have wisdom to share with others in the sector, whether they are new or experienced practitioners. These interviews became **Advice for Surf Therapy Practitioners,** which collects their advice into a masterclass in wisdom on items ranging from how to get funding, how to keep the passion to help others burn bright, how to grow a surf therapy organization from the ground up and much more.

And finally, while this book is a collection of stories—as is any story so focused on the human experience—I want first and foremost to ensure that these stories led to action, whether it's volunteering, getting involved, or starting your own surf therapy movement. This is why, in **Surf Therapy Resource Guide,** I've compiled a list of surf therapy organizations around the world (connected with ISTO) so that anyone can get connected to the surf therapy industry.

I hope this book entertains you so that, despite the addictive social media algorithms that beckon us, you can't stop flipping its pages. I hope it educates you—as it did me—on the growing body of evidence of how surf therapy is therapeutic. And, most of all, I hope the stories inside—the stories of struggles and triumph—inspire you about how far a human will go to help another in need.

1

THE ORIGINS OF SURF THERAPY

hile there is no definitive history that tells us surf therapy was used by ancient cultures—the term "surf therapy" itself is exclusive to the 21st century—we do have interesting hints that are worth examining.

For centuries, many cultures around the world feared the sea, a massive and unpredictable body that stretched to the horizon. Tales of angry gods, along with out-of-this world-creatures who trapped its victims underneath the salty surface abounded.

Though there were many cultures who feared the sea, some respected it—and lived in harmony with its unpredictability. One of those cultures was the Native Hawaiians, who left us a hint that surf therapy may have been practiced.

This hint comes from *The Epic Tale of Hi'iakaikapoliopele*. The ancient story, which was translated in this century, chronicles the use of surfing as a modality of healing.

In Ancient Hawaiian lore, Hi'iaka is known as the Hawaiian patron goddess of hula dancers, chant, sorcery, and medicine, and is the younger sister of Pele, the Goddess of Fire and Volcanoes.

In the tale, Hi'iaka is sent by Pele, the Goddess of Fire and Volcanoes, on a journey from Hawaii's Big Island across the Hawaiian Island chain to Kauai to bring back Lohi'au, a mortal chieftain, because Pele favored him.[11]

When Hi'iaka arrived in Kauai, she discovered that Lohi'au had died. Instead of taking it as a finality, Hi'iaka uses chants, prayers, and medicine, which temporarily brings his soul back into his body; but to finish the job, she takes him surfing:

> *"As the rays of the sun shimmered upon the surface of the sea, Hi'iaka beckoned the waves to rise. A great gust of wind suddenly struck and an enormous swell arose, billowed up, and towered steeply, as Hi'iaka spurred on Lohi'au. He flew like a wave-flitting 'akihi bird as he perched on the crest of the wave. Hi'iaka followed, alighting on the crest ... Hi'iaka's skirt became a surfboard for Lohi'au, while Hi'iaka's chest, her whole body, actually, became her board to ride the waves. As he surfed, Lohi'au could see that everything about him was in peak condition. All of his physical strength had come back to him, just as it was before. Lohi'au surfed the wave, shifting his stance, coasting forward over the broad part of the break and moving back along the narrows, gliding back and forth. ... Hi'iaka stood upon the surface of the water with her skirt of pahapaha seaweed and mokila grass fluttering behind her. And Lohi'au tried out every possible surfing stance, each of which he could perform with ease. They continued on until the uplands of Ha'ena lay clearly before them and its populace saw these three people standing in the curl of the wave. They surfed along and cut right in front of where Kahuanui and the rest were sitting. From there, the wave broke and swept back out to sea. And now they surfed it back out, riding atop the shoulder of the*

wave. The shore filled with shouting voices of the people, their roar echoing against the sea cliffs. Nothing could compare to the beauty of this surfing."[12]

What I found so fascinating is that, in this Native Hawaiian story, the healing process consisted of prayers, medicine, and surfing—the last of which was used to bring Lohi'au back to full strength. Hi'iaka—the goddess of medicine—knew the power of surfing, and when it was used alongside other healing modalities, it had a powerful and therapeutic effect.

Does this story definitively communicate that Native Hawaiians used surfing as a part of the healing process? Dr. Puakea Nogelmeier, the story's translator, and the Professor Emeritus of Hawaiian Language at the University of Hawai'i at Mānoa told me that it doesn't.

"Surfing is certainly used as part of the healing process to revive Lohi'au, but it's unique. I can't think of another instance where surfing is used like this," he said.

What makes it so difficult to analyze whether or not Native Hawaiians used surf therapy is that we're looking at it from a 21st century, Westernized perspective.

"Hawaiians have always had a healing relationship with the ocean," said Dr. Kau'i Baumhofer Merritt, an Assistant Professor of Indigenous Health Sciences at the University of Hawai'i - West O'ahu. She explained that there likely were no connections between surfing and therapy at the time because Native Hawaiians didn't separate the two as we do today. Surfing was a mental, physical, and spiritual activity—an activity that excited and healed—all wrapped up in one.

For Kris Primacio, CEO of the International Surf Therapy Organization (ISTO), we can't draw historical conclusions from these hints, but we can draw personal ones. "In surf therapy, surfing alone is not considered the same as surf therapy," she told me. By the International

Surf Therapy Organization's definition, surf therapy is "The use of surfing as a vehicle for delivering intentional, inclusive, population-specific, and evidenced-based therapeutic structures to promote psychological, physical, and psychosocial well-being. By ISTO's definition of surf therapy, we don't have any evidence that people intentionally came together to promote well-being. But I firmly believe that Native Hawaiians had already been experiencing the therapeutic benefits of the ocean and surfing centuries before it was officially recognized."

ᑫᑫᑫ

In contrast, we know the first instance of surf therapy by the International Surf Therapy Organization's specific definition, took place on July 3, 1986, at Ventura County Line, where Ted Silverberg and a group of surfer friends took blind children surfing.

Ted, a surfer in his late 20s, owned and operated Paradise Surfing Lessons in Malibu, California. The Braille Institute of Los Angeles contacted him and explained their summer program, where they gave their visually impaired students a chance to experience sports that they otherwise wouldn't have the chance to, including rock climbing, waterskiing, camping, and more. They wanted to know if Ted would take them surfing.

"They just asked me if I could teach some blind children to surf, and I told them there was only one way to find out," he said in an interview with the Los Angeles Times.[13]

But before the surfing event, Ted wanted to gain a greater understanding for the kids and their swimming ability. He loaded up a bunch of longboards on top of his car and drove south from Malibu to the Braille Institute in Los Angeles. Once there, he placed a surfboard in the pool, sat on it, and told the kids, one at a time, to swim out to him. They could swim well and could balance on the board well with Ted.

But he noticed something troublesome: each of the children would jump off the board and swim to the side of the pool, knowing where safety was based off memory. In the unfamiliar ocean, they wouldn't have this ability. If a child fell off the board, he or she could start swimming directly out to sea without realizing it.

To prepare for this, Ted and a few surfer friends he recruited to help as volunteers went to Malibu's Surfrider Beach. There, Ted paddled and tried to catch waves with his eyes closed and realized just how challenging it would be to do so blind.

So, on July 3, Ted, and a few other volunteer surf instructors arrived at County Line. "The reason we were there is because there were no lifeguards or police who might tell us we couldn't do it at that location," Ted told me. The children from the Braille Institute arrived, about 20 in the ages of 5–18. Most were legally blind, and a few others were completely blind.

Since most, if not all, of the participants knew nothing of the ocean and had never even been to the beach, Ted and the instructors first explained waves and the tide—Ted cupped his hand in the shape of a wave and allowed the participants to feel it to help prove the point—and then taught the students how to stand up on a board. The surf experience would be a 1:1 ratio, with Ted and the instructors paddling for waves, and telling the children when to stand and enjoy the ride.

What happened next was hard to describe without bringing tears to Ted's eyes. He remembers a child feeling the saltwater spray from a wave in his face and saying 'wow, it tastes salty!' He remembers a child touching seaweed for the first time and not knowing what it was. He remembers the facial expressions as they caught waves.

"It was the greatest experience I ever had," he said.

Having had such a profound experience taking the blind participants surfing, Ted decided to take the participants surfing again. He had no idea at the time what it would grow into.

Ted rallied sponsors like Body Glove, who donated wetsuits, and BZ Surfboards, who donated 9 feet long, 5 inch thick boards. By their second year, they had more than a dozen sponsors, including Zuma Jay Surfboards, Mugsea Actionwear, Body Glove Wetsuits, Astrodeck, Aloegator, Casio, Vuarnet and more.

He also rallied more surf instructor volunteers—Todd Roberts, Jamie Brisick, Mikke Pierson, Tim Ball, Jeff Edgar, Bob Terry and Casey Fleming—and for training, he took them out to Surfrider Beach to help them understand what the kids would experience.

Mikke Pierson remembers that in order to prepare, they each paddled around at Surfrider Beach with their eyes closed to try and understand what the participants would be experiencing.

In the mid-1980s, Ted and other surfers didn't have surf forecasting sites at their fingertips, so he relied on friend Sean Collins, the founder of Surfline, to tell him when the waves would be not too big, but not too small for taking the kids surfing.

For the next events, instead of the County Line, Ted decided to hold events at Surfrider Beach. But that presented a problem: with a crowded and heavily localized lineup, the risk of a volunteer and child getting run into or run over was extremely high.

Before the time of permits that would clear the spot, they decided to get creative. Ted asked some locals to block and keep the waters clear so that no one would get hurt.

"Taking over Malibu was a heroic feat," Ted said.

Mikke told me that while some surfers respected it, a few didn't. "I had taken off on a wave, and our water patrol was trying to stop an old guy on a longboard who didn't give a damn what we were doing, and we all collided. Tumbling upside down with a blind participant and we're all in the white water...I popped up and didn't see him. I was in a complete panic. I found him under the board. I remember thinking 'wow, this is intense.' This is real life."

"People were mind blown that legally blind kids would have the guts to do this," Ted said. "And I agreed with them."

"One kid kept saying, 'I'm not scared, I'm not scared, I'm not scared," Silverberg recalled. "I asked him why he kept saying it, and he said, 'Everybody tells me I have a fear of everything, and I have to keep saying I'm not afraid.' He was great out there. He loved it."[14]

"There's no doubt that they're scared when they first try it, but we try and reassure them," said Steve Lackey, assistant director at the Braille Institute's youth center. "The goal is to let them overcome their fears."[15]

When Ted and I first spoke, he communicated that he had a trove of archives that put all of these memories into photos. After flying into Kona, located on the Hawaii's Big Island, I met him at his beautiful property perched on a mountainside with endless views of the Pacific on the horizon.

Ted began pulling photos out of his storage area and putting them on the kitchen table for me to examine. The photos brought tears to my eyes: a much younger version of Ted, with a BZ surfboard under his arm, holding hands with a blind girl wearing a green Body Glove rash guard and walking her back from a surf session; A yearbook style photo of him, sitting with dozens of blind children at the Braille Institute, holding a surfboard and absolutely beaming; him going down the line of a wave with a participant.

Amongst the photos, I found an excerpt from Surfer Magazine, circa 1989, that read:

> *"A familiar scene, with a twist: As young Brian Goldblatt Grips the nose of a soft surfboard, Paradise Surfing Lessons instructor Ted Silverberg turns into a small right at First Point Malibu. If Brian looks more excited than the average first time grommet, that's because he's blind, and is getting stoked on the*

pure sensuous feeling of riding a cracking, fast wave through cool waters on a hot summer day. On Thursday, July 20, Brian and 20 of his schoolmates from the Los Angeles Braille Institute spent a Thursday afternoon in 3–4 foot surf at Malibu with Silverberg, Bob Terry, Todd Roberts and Mike Pierson. As cheers went up from the beach, each of the kids had a chance to experience something that would otherwise be off-limits to them. Most of the beginners were scared at first, as they tried to identify and sort out the cacophony of sounds, smells and feelings bombarding them from the ocean and the beach. However, Brian's after-session dance is indicative of how he enjoyed the experience, and all his schoolmates responded similarly, as they added surf stoke to their inventory of new sensations."[16]

But the benefits were not isolated to the participants. The volunteers also experienced an unusual feeling of stoke. "When you're done with that kind of day, you're so amped," Mikke told me. "As much as you give back, you get more in return. I'll never forget that stoke of working with the kids. It was a mind-blowing feeling."

Both Ted and Mikke told me "It was never a thought that we were the first." They didn't think about growing it into an organization. They just wanted to lend a helping hand.

Along with giving back, Ted explained that the perception of surfers in the 1980s wasn't the best. Giving back could help this perception, and "show surfing had class, prestige, and was a good sport," he said.

After 2000, Ted stopped doing the events, the tides of life pulling him and the other surf volunteers in different directions.

While digging through Ted's archives, I found a typed letter he wrote after the first event that summarized the essence of what had transpired. Ted didn't know it at the time, but it included an inspirational charge to the surf therapy community that would organically grow years later. It read:

*"I would like to challenge my fellow surfers to start a new era
by each of us giving a little bit back to the sport that is such
an important part of our lives. I challenge us to progress and
promote surfing as the world's healthiest sport! ... The fact that
my day shared with the children of the Braille Institute received
newspaper and TV coverage made me proud of the image my
sport was projecting to the world. The true essence of surfing
was never more prevalent than on that day when a group of
people got together, shared the innate beauty of the beach and
respect for the ocean and a good time was had by all. If I could
teach only one thing to all surfers, it would be "to give a little
bit back" to surfing."[17]*

eee

Over the next two decades, the surf therapy sector grew organically,
driven by the same qualities that drove Ted Silverberg—a passion to
help others in need.

After seeing the benefits of taking his child, diagnosed with autism,
surfing, Israel "Izzy" Paskowitz founded Surfer's Healing in 1996—the
original surf camp for children on the autism spectrum that primarily
operates out of Southern California.

In 1998, Danny Cortazzo wanted to give back to those with special
needs in Santa Cruz, California, through surfing, and founded Ride
a Wave Foundation. Wanting to take participants with cerebral palsy
out to surf, Danny and his team made what's considered one of the
first adaptive surfboard the sector had seen and used it for therapeutic
purposes.

Years after falling headfirst into a shallow sandbar while surfing and
suffering instant paralysis, Jesse Billauer founded Life Rolls On in 2001
to help others with paralysis surf.

In 2005, the Jimmy Miller Memorial Foundation introduced surf therapy to both underprivileged and abused children in the Los Angeles community to honor the life and legacy of Jimmy Miller, who served as a L.A. County Lifeguard for fifteen years—most of those years spent in Manhattan Beach.

By 2010—when I experienced my surf therapy event in Florida—surf therapy itself was not only taking place on both of America's coasts; the same year, a group of volunteers took children and young adults with mental health disorders surfing in England; in 2011, surf therapy was being utilized to take children in poverty-stricken townships in South Africa into the sea.

Nearly a decade after Ted's events concluded, surf therapy was more prevalent, yes, but in reality, it was isolated to particular needs amongst specific populations.

Then, in 2017, something happened that would serve as the catalyst for the sector to grow. Waves for Change, a surf therapy organization based in Cape Town, South Africa, had received a grant to grow not just their program, but the sector as a whole. Eight organizations from around the world sent practitioners to Cape Town. From the outside, it may not have looked like much—a group of surfers talking about surf therapy—but it was the most significant meeting in the history of the surf therapy sector to date.

One person present was Kris Primacio, an energetic and sweet woman with Native Hawaiian roots who, at the time, served as the Program Manager for The Jimmy Miller Memorial Foundation. Kris understood the power of surf therapy firsthand.

She began surfing in 2011, six months after her father was diagnosed with cancer. "I sought the ocean's healing powers to turn off the heartache of watching my father endure the relentless stages of terminal cancer," she told me. "The ocean, God bless her, embraced my heartache like nothing else could have. I discovered what so many people already knew—surfing gets you into a flow state. During that time, mixing my saltwater tears with the saltwater in the ocean was extremely comforting. The ocean healed me, and it's a place where I still find refuge. It feels like a hug when you're immersed in the arms of the ocean."

For five days, the group, including Kris, shared, brainstormed, laughed, cried, and differed on how to grow the sector. The result was the creation of an international body that would serve as the meeting point for all surf therapy organizations, from past to present and future: the International Surf Therapy Organization (ISTO).

The goal of ISTO is simple: bring together surf therapy organizations, share methods, facilitate research, and promote better practices so more people can safely and inclusively experience the healing powers of surfing.

A mere nine months later, in 2018, 35 individuals representing 15 surf therapy organizations gathered in Jeffrey's Bay for the second annual ISTO conference.

One of the main discussion points was the organization's growth—which required someone at the helm. Kris was chosen.

"One year after we officially launched, I was appointed CEO of ISTO. It was exciting and intimidating all at once," Kris said.[18] "By harnessing the power of partnership, we know we can make bigger waves. We are expanding surf therapy awareness worldwide by increasing the research, [as well as] developing and sharing our practices."

According to Kris, ISTO exists "to provide access to resources and connect practitioners in meaningful ways to learn from one another."

Through this, new practitioners have unlimited help and inspiration through online monthly working groups, quarterly webinars, and annual conferences—none of which existed before ISTO.

Collectively, ISTO decided upon the theme of "Go Far Go Together," a shortened version of an African proverb. "What we found is that very few organizations spoke to one another or even knew other organizations existed," Kris told me. "It felt like we were better together."

In 2019, ISTO hosted a conference that showed just how far they had grown in just two years: 50 surf therapy organizations, 40 guest speakers (myself included to discuss *Waves of Healing*), and, in total, a little under 300 people.

To be a member of ISTO, you must do two things: first, contribute to surf therapy, and second, contribute to data around surf therapy. One of ISTO's most significant achievements to date is the latter.

"Evidence and exposure bring validation," Kris says. "Our vision is universal acceptance through prescription. We can't do that without data."[19]

Before ISTO, less than 20 surf therapy publications had been published.[20]

In 2020, the *Global Journal of Community Psychology Practice* released the First-Ever Special Issue Dedicated to Surf Therapy Research Around the World. The Special Issue featured eight-peer reviewed articles, including 39 authors, researchers, scholars, students, practitioners, clinicians, and ISTO contributing members. The idea to collectively submit research articles to an academic journal was made during the ISTO 2018 conference in Jeffrey's Bay by ISTO Advisor Gregor Sarkisian. The issue also included a comprehensive scoping review yielding 29 papers.

"This Special Focus Issue on Surf Therapy Around the Globe includes the most comprehensive collection of research on surf therapy," said Gregor Sarkisian, Ph.D., who teaches psychology at Antioch University in Los Angeles. "It includes empirical research on eight surf therapy programs delivered across six countries—Ireland, the Netherlands, Portugal, South Africa, the United Kingdom, and the United States of America—serving diverse populations, including youth with disabilities, vulnerable youth, active-duty military service members and military veterans."[21]

"That journal alone tripled the research in surf therapy," Kris told me. "I am stoked about the growing amount of data in the surf therapy industry and feel fortunate to be a witness to it all. I believe that surf therapy will become widely recognized and appreciated. It's exciting to think that we will have been a part of its early development."

Some of the study's findings included:

- Surf therapy resulted in improvements in physical fitness, self-confidence, social development, behavior and sleep, and reduced levels of anxiety for youth with disabilities.[22]
- Surf therapy improved self-concept, emotional regulation and social competencies of children and youth in need of social and emotional support. In addition to this, participants also experienced re-engagement with school, and decreases in behavioral problems reported post-intervention.[23]
- Surf therapy helped active-duty military service members decrease their symptoms of depression, anxiety, and PTSD. In addition to this, an active-duty military service member, surfing was found to have the ability to provide an alternative form of pain management.[24]
- Surf therapy provided respite from the symptoms of PTSD, in addition to decreased stress levels, depressive symptoms and use of narcotics, and an increase in feelings of self-efficacy for a population of military veterans.[25]
- Surf therapy improved the body image, self-esteem, and self-compassion of a young adult population of cancer survivors. In addition, the participants reported decreases in self-reported depressive symptoms/depression as well as decreased feelings of alienation.[26]
- Many more surprising, data-proven findings on the results of surf therapy.

"This recognition validates our efforts to bring together a level of collaboration and medical legitimacy that hasn't been seen before in surf therapy," Kris told me. "Data is the new healthcare currency. Protecting and growing it is vital for systematic change, so we have prioritized advancing research."

While practitioners like Kris know that surf therapy works personally and amongst others, this never-before-seen collection of data helped further validate surf therapy's effectiveness to academia.

What has also helped grow surf therapy's presence in academia is the first-ever Ph.D. in surf therapy—an impressive title held by Scotsman Dr. Jamie Marshall, Research Fellow at Edinburgh Napier University.

Like many key players in the industry, Jamie first experienced how therapeutic surfing could be—and wanted to share it with others.

"When I look back on my life, a career in surf therapy seems inevitable," he told me. "When I was at school, I struggled with some significant bullying which definitely affected my own mental health. When I was about 15, I got invited on a trip through the school and experienced surfing for the first time. I paddled into that first wave and all of that washed away. All the anecdotes you hear about surfing being therapeutic was true for me in that moment. Surfing gave me an identity and a feeling that no bully could take away."

Jamie was asked to volunteer with the Wave Project, a UK based surf therapy program founded in 2010, and for the first time, he saw the effects that surfing had on participants with autism. "Seeing the joy these guys and girls had, it was just infectious," he said.

Witnessing how surfing was therapeutic for himself and others made Jamie curious. "Seeing these big changes that happen to young people, to veterans…when you say it out loud it's unbelievable… people speaking again after going mute or being free from flashbacks. I was really struck by this when I was running the program [the Wave Project's Scotland program], I wanted to know what was going on."

One of the volunteers Jamie worked with was a lecturer at the University of Edinburgh in Scotland, and the person recommended

Jamie to a Masters program where he could study physical activity's impact on mental health, if not surfing specifically.

Jamie said that his Masters research led to "some theories" about surfing's therapeutic properties, but he needed to go deeper—the impetus behind beginning his PhD.

"I've experienced people saying that surf therapy wasn't evidence based, and that mirrors what other surf therapy practitioners have experienced...'You aren't serious about helping people, you just want to go surfing.' The ultimate response to that is that I surfed less during the write up of my PhD than any other point in my surfing life! It was complete irony."

Jamie examined a range of populations around the world, including "military veterans in the USA, youth in post conflict Liberia, and youth at-risk-of or with mental health diagnosis in Australia."[27] He compiled his findings in *A Global Exploration of Programme Theory within Surf Therapy*. In the abstract, Jamie summarized his conclusions by noting the growing understanding and evidence behind surf therapy:

> *"The findings from the current research programme have presented an original and significant contribution to knowledge around programme theory within surf therapy and mental health. Taken together, all these conclusions make significant contributions to surf therapy's aim of becoming a trusted, prescribed, and standard means of care in supporting global mental health."[28]*

Today, Jamie remains the pioneer of a doctorate in surf therapy—leading the way for other academic studies to follow. In addition, as a board member for ISTO, he is in constant contact with surf therapy practitioners from around the world—a community that has recently grown even larger.

ISTO's growth has reached new heights up to the present time. As of 2023, they are engaged with 133 surf therapy organizations around the world—more than a 1550 percent growth in surf therapy programs.

Regarding where ISTO is headed, they're promoting surf therapy with a goal—"Inclusive access to evidence-based, safe surf therapy worldwide." Kris told me. She referenced the Wave Project—a UK-based surf therapy organization that has several programs within its organization that is funded by the National Health Service (NHS) and, therefore, the first surf therapy program recognized financially by a healthcare institution. "If more institutions acknowledge the effectiveness of surf therapy and provide funding, it can lead to the creation of more programs. This, in turn, can ensure that more people in need have access to this beneficial form of therapy. Here in the US, we need more RCTs (randomized controlled trials). Programming must go through all the checks and balances. Surf therapy will undoubtedly be added to the list of alternative treatment methods for mental health, but we have a long way to go."

Today, ISTO and its global coalition of surf therapy organizations have one goal with surf therapy, and it's the same goal that Ted Silverberg and his friends had in the 1980s, and the same goal that Hi'iaka had in *The Epic Tale of Hi'ikaikapoliopele*: to use surfing as a means of healing.

2

WAR, PTSD & SURF THERAPY FOR MILITARY SERVICE MEMBERS

When you think of PTSD, usually what comes to mind first is war—a battlefield, explosions, seeing death before your very eyes. Some Military service members return home with physical wounds; others return with mental wounds. In many cases, it's both. As a result of the 9/11 attacks in the United States, the War on Terror began at the start of the century—and no one could foresee both the physical toll for those who made the ultimate sacrifice for their country and the mental toll for those who would return home. Rates of PTSD and other mental ailments skyrocketed among this population—and so did suicide.

I spoke with two organizations on both of America's coasts to learn more about how they are using surfing to help active duty service members and veterans heal from the traumas of war and active duty—and, in many instances, how they are preventing PTSD from taking a life.

But for surf therapy to continue to serve as an alternative form of treatment, there must be evidence-based data showing its efficacy. I also spoke with three women who pioneered research among this population—and laid the foundation for surf therapy research for the sector to follow.

$$\mathcal{eee}$$

The story begins with Carly M. Rogers, OTD, OTR/L who is known as the "mother of surf therapy," but formally carries the title "Ocean Therapy Consultant."

A Southern California native and lifelong surfer, Carly became a Los Angeles County Ocean Lifeguard in 1994, and by 1997, she also served as a W.A.T.E.R. Program outreach instructor teaching public safety in Los Angeles County. Because of this, it was routine for her to teach children and young adults the joys of the sea, along with its dangers.

But one of these experiences was far from routine—it changed her life.

One day, she led inner city children, some of whom had special needs, to the beach to teach them about ocean safety. One of the participants was a young boy confined to a wheelchair. After his wheelchair rolled onto the sand, his eyes were focused on the ocean, and he began squirming to get out of the chair and into the sea.

"I could barely get his seatbelt off, and he dove out in the sand and started crawling towards the water," Carly said.[29] "Instantly, as it does now, my skin lit up and I said oh my gosh, we have to take these kids surfing!"

She soon found the field of occupational therapy, and attended University of Southern California to obtain her Masters. As part of her program, she conceptualized what a surf therapy program would look like and thought about its overall goal.

"What was the goal? Was it just to learn to surf? It was so much more than that," Carly said. "I thought about that child in the wheelchair, it was self-efficacy in its purest form, what Albert Bandura describes as our personal belief in our ability to achieve a goal."[30]

As she was finishing her Masters, tragedy struck that would intertwine Carly's concept of a surf therapy program to a present day need in the local community.

Carly received word that Jimmy Miller, a lifeguard who mentored Carly, and someone she held in high esteem, took his own life. Jimmy had served as an L.A. County Lifeguard for fifteen years, and through his surf camp called "Pure Surfing Experience" and later, "Camp Surf," had taught countless people to surf, held surf contests, and personified showing others the powers of the sea through giving back.

In 2004, Jimmy had sustained a shoulder injury that kept him out of the water. That, coupled with the "rapid onset of undiagnosed mental illness"[31] resulted in him taking his own life, and many of Jimmy's friends and family believe that had he been able to surf, the outcome could have been different.

In 2005, the Jimmy Miller Memorial Foundation (JMMF) was founded to continue his legacy of sharing "his pure love of surfing and the ocean with those suffering from mental and physical illness around the world."[32]

This new surf therapy organization needed a program, and Carly had her recent work to serve as exactly that—her title became the "Director of Programs" for the surf therapy organization that focused on "serving underprivileged children in Los Angeles."

While there was no literature that showed the efficacy of surf therapy, the immediate results that Carly and JMMF saw spoke volumes.

"The results were beyond our wildest expectations and remarkable. As one clinician stated, 'These children have experienced such trauma that there are no positive memories for them to

refer to. You have created positive memories for them that will serve them for a lifetime. You have inspired the very core of who they are and what they can accomplish."[33]

In 2006, a friend of Carly's had the idea to take the JMMF program to returning veterans from Iraq and Afghanistan at Camp Pendleton, a Marine Corps Base in Southern California. The goal behind the effort was to see if surfing could "rinse off the symptoms of PTSD."[34]

Yearlong conversations with both the Pentagon and military command followed—Carly remembers being told that surfing was too dangerous for veterans, and that there was no way doctors would actually let them surf. Despite the pushback, Carly and her team were invited to Camp Pendleton to do a pilot program with the Wounded Warrior Battalion.

At the beach, Carly saw surfing have an immediate effect from a therapist lens. Initially, there was little eye contact and interest from the participants; the scene was quiet and tense. Once they were in the water surfing, the scene had transformed: participants were smiling, cheering, and laughing, and excitement filled the Pacific air.

"Oh, my God, our Marines are talking about how they feel," said the lieutenant who had approved the experiment. "They don't talk. Ever."[35]

The feedback she received during a discussion session post surfing reinforced the therapeutic benefits she had seen. One participant said "this could save my life. I feel finally alive!"[36]

Another participant said: "Oh my gosh, I haven't laughed or felt so good in forever. This is incredible, who knew surfing could be therapeutic?!"[37]

And, most powerful of all, one participant, after making it beyond the breaking waves, started splashing the water while exclaiming, "this is curing my PTSD!"[38]

What was also powerful were the lingering effects of surfing into the night. Because the session took place over two days, the group went to sleep, and the next morning, several participants reported that they slept far longer that night than they had in recent memory, sleep disturbance being a common symptom of those diagnosed with PTSD.

The command staff of the Wounded Warrior Battalion saw the effects as well. "The change at the barracks is visceral. The Marines come back from (Surf Therapy) sessions with actual smiles on their faces. This is something we have not been able to provide through traditional therapy."[39]

After this initial success, JMMF created a veterans program in 2007 to provide a safe and therapeutic environment for veterans to experience the healing powers of the sea.

Carly went back to school to study the effects of the program. One of her first findings was that not only did veterans have decreased reported symptoms of PTSD and depression; they also had prominent attendance rates—75 percent of the participants traveled 20 miles to attend and came to three or more sessions.[40]

Carly also had the groundbreaking realization that surfing is, in a way, the antithesis of PTSD. She said:

> *"The three main symptoms of PTSD ... The first is isolation or avoidance of preferred activities. The second is a re-experiencing trauma in the form of flashbacks and nightmares, the trauma never leaves them. The third is hyper arousal or hyper vigilance where they're constantly in a state of fight or flight. In surfing, instead of avoidance, it's complete engagement. Your senses are aware, your body is aware, you're present. Instead of re-experiencing the trauma, like I said, you're completely present in the moment. So many participants said, 'I wasn't thinking about anything but being in the water.' Hyper arousal,*

of course, there's an adrenaline rush with surfing as one partic-
ipant stated so poignantly, he said, 'In combat you wait and
wait and then you engage in an intense firefight for your life. In
surfing, you wait and wait and then you engage in a pure and
natural adrenaline rush. I never knew how beautiful mother
nature could be.'"[41]

Carly's findings were published in what was regarded as the first study on surf therapy: *High-Intensity Sports for Posttraumatic Stress Disorder and Depression: Feasibility Study of Ocean Therapy With Veterans of Operation Enduring Freedom and Operation Iraqi Freedom.* The study found:

"Participants reported clinically meaningful improvement in
PTSD symptom severity and in depressive symptoms. The results
of this small, uncontrolled study suggest that a sports-oriented
occupational therapy intervention has potential as a feasible
adjunct intervention for veterans seeking mental health treat-
ment for symptoms of PTSD."[42]

In the coming years, JMMF's veteran program helped thousands of veterans experience the therapeutic nature of surf therapy.

In time, the Foundation itself grew to coordinate up to 50 surf therapy sessions each year—veterans included—for a wide range of populations.

Carly's "mother of surf therapy" moniker is no exaggeration. Not only did she put one of the first surf therapy program concepts on paper; her study served as the foundational piece of surf therapy research in academia. Both of these achievements became the solid foundation that the surf therapy sector then built upon in the years to come.

In 2017, she was a vital voice in the development of the International Surf Therapy Organization (ISTO). Today, she still serves as an Ocean Therapy Consultant, often re-telling the story of witnessing the boy, confined to a wheelchair, crawling towards the water—and how we all can benefit from the healing powers of the sea.

♻ ♻ ♻

In 2008, Betty Michalewicz-Kragh, an exercise physiologist at Naval Medical Center San Diego, was tasked with providing rehabilitation with combat-injured service members, coping from polytrauma, amputations, PTSD, Traumatic Brain Injury (TBI), and more.

One of the first combat injured service members that Betty met was a soldier, who had lost both an arm and a leg in Operation Iraqi Freedom. When Betty conducted her assessment, the service member told her that he was from Hawaii. When Betty asked what physical activity he would like to get engaged with, the soldier replied that he wished he would surf again some day. That was 2008, and the concept of surf therapy did not exist yet. However, seeing how important surfing was to his morale, Betty believed that surfing could help him, and decided to make it happen. She went to work helping him condition for it, such as swimming, building muscle strength and endurance, and even practicing maneuvering a surfboard in a pool.

Betty spent her nights researching adaptive surf therapy, a subject on which there was very little literature at the time. Her mission was to get just this service member back in the water, and once that had happened, she believed it would be mission accomplished.

"I never thought it would grow into a weekly, reoccurring surf therapy program," Betty told me over the phone, the sounds of a military medical center echoing through the speaker.

To say the program grew is an understatement. More Naval Medical Center San Diego combat-injured patients became interested in surfing, lining up to get their medical clearances and make their medical appointments for this unique form of treatment. Betty calls the fact that surf therapy was a formal, scheduled medical appointment "groundbreaking," and very helpful too in setting the surf therapy modality for success: "Many times people who are coping with depression and/or PTSD, want to be left alone. Often just the thought of being out on a crowded beach is overwhelming," Betty told me. "But when you are in the military and you have a 'medical appointment,' it is your responsibility to attend that medical appointment, and it is your 'place of accountability.' The fact that it was a medical appointment was a key to the program's success," she said. She remembers many times when patients would come to her after their surf session with a huge smile on their face and tell her that coming to a busy hot beach was the last thing they wanted to do when they woke up depressed in the morning, yet they were so glad they came.

For the next 13 years, Betty took wounded, injured, and ill service members surfing every Thursday at Del Mar Beach, along with the help of many community volunteers. The NMCSD surf therapy program was supported by the Del Mar Beach lifeguards, who kept a watchful eye to ensure the surfers' safety, and by many other nonprofit organizations such as "Armed Services YMCA," "Semper Fi Fund," "Challenged Athlete Foundation," and many more.

The first year's NMCSD Surf Therapy program patient population was mainly OEF and OIF combat injured service members. Many of the wounded warriors at that time were amputees: Betty recalls realizing, while talking to six Marines, patients—surfers, wounded warriors—"that there were only five legs between all these six Marines."

A study, published in 2011, called "*Surf Medicine: Surfing as a Means of Therapy for Combat-Related Polytrauma*," revealed just how therapeutic these surf sessions were.

The study examined a "21-year-old active duty US Army soldier who had been exposed to a blast injury that culminated in a bilateral transfemoral amputation, severe burn injuries, traumatic brain injury (TBI), mild depression, and severe pain. After multiple surgeries, the patient was treated with physical therapy for strength and balance, opiates for pain, and psychotherapy for acute care. Although the patient's symptoms improved significantly from his baseline, he continued to experience severe symptoms, including limited use of prosthetic limbs; use of morphine, tramadol, and oxycodone; and residual symptoms of decline in well-being."[43]

The results of surf therapy on this participant were profound:

> "After six months in this program, engaging once a week for three hours per session for six months, the patient reported significant progress. His improvement in balance exceeded that of his peers with the same condition. He was the only patient at that time with bilateral transfemoral amputations who was able to walk on two prostheses as a primary means of movement. He was able to discontinue narcotics (Figure 1). His depression completely resolved, and he reported complete relief from symptoms on days during which he went surfing. He also reported that participation in the surf clinic had significantly improved his general well-being and stress level."[44]

"We always told patients of Naval Medical Center San Diego the idea of the program was for them to find out if this modality of care is beneficial for them. And if it is, the goal was for them to be able to surf safely and independently to utilize this modality safely and independently," Betty said.

Betty watched in real time as surfing helped patients of the Naval Medical Center San Diego, like Jose Martinez.

"It pretty much saved my life. I don't think I can put it any lighter than that," said Jose Martinez, an Army veteran who lost both his legs, his right arm, a finger on his left hand, and internal organs due to an IED explosion as he was on foot patrol during Operation Enduring Freedom in 2012 in Kandahar, Afghanistan.

In 2014, while Martinez was recovering at Naval Medical Center San Diego, Betty asked him about getting in the water and swimming. "Being a triple amputee, I told her no," Martinez said. "But she knew how much being in the water could help me."

Martinez told Betty that if he could have his colostomy bag reversed, he would give it a go. Months later, Martinez was true to his word and tried to swim with Betty monitoring him.

At first, swimming was difficult: "I could crawl faster than I could swim," Martinez told me—but driven by the fact that swimming would help his core, which could help him walk again and his overall health, Martinez didn't give up.

Seeing his progress in the pool, Betty asked if he wanted to try surfing.

"My first thought was I only have 1 arm...how am I going to surf?" he said.

One Thursday morning at Del Mar beach, he remembers his first wave. After being pushed by a volunteer in whitewash, Martinez felt "euphoria". He was instantly hooked.

"The more I surfed, the more I felt myself again," he said. "And the more I felt free."

Martinez credits surfing with not only giving him that euphoria, but also helping to mitigate other forms of prescribed therapy. "I'm supposed to be on all kinds of painkillers, all kinds of depression pills, but I don't take any of them. Surfing is my depression pill," he said.

Along with serving as the Vice President and CoFounder of Four Seasons Fighters, an organization dedicated to helping service men and women, Martinez has pursued surfing to the point of representing Team USA at the Parasurfing Championships.

As the War on Terror drew to a close—where US service men and women fought in both Iraq and Afghanistan post 9/11—the needs of veterans changed from physical rehabilitation to mental rehabilitation. The military saw a 65 percent increase in mental-health diagnoses among active-duty personnel between 2001 and 2011, according to a 2013 study conducted by the Congressional Research Service. More specifically, cases of PTSD increased by 650 percent, and more than 900,000 individuals were diagnosed with at least one mental disorder during that decade.[45]

But Betty told me that these events didn't disqualify surf therapy. "As we realized the mental benefits of surf therapy, we adjusted the mission to NMCSD current patient population, so NMCSD SURF THERAPY program remained relevant as the war wound down."

"We took care of 24 patients on a weekly basis, and people told me it saved their lives," Betty said.

What is most surprising to Betty, looking back, is the cost of treatment. "It touched thousands of lives, providing physical, mental, spiritual, and emotional benefits, including community re-integration for the wounded warriors as well as introduction of the troops to the community," she said. "Yet the cost was so minimal thanks to the community support."

Betty's original goal was to help one soldier experience surfing again, and she certainly accomplished that mission. She also accomplished helping many other service members experience surf therapy—and make tremendous contributions to the growing body of its evidence.

eee

Kristen Walter calls her introduction into surf therapy "purely serendipitous." In 2013, she relocated from Ohio to San Diego and through her new position, served as a volunteer at the Department of Veterans Affairs (VA)-sponsored National Veterans Summer Sports Clinic (NVSSC)—which offers "adventure sports to post 9/11 veterans engaged in a rehabilitation (or other) treatment program, or whose current rehabilitation goals would benefit from the value of adaptive summer sports." One of those "adventure sports" is surfing.

After arriving at La Jolla Shores, Kristen volunteered by keeping an eye on participants and instructors alike to ensure safety and ensure that surfboards made it back to the beach instead of being pulled out into the endless Pacific Ocean.

She had a front row seat to the surfing, yes, but also the therapeutic aspect of surfing on display—and it made her curious.

"I'm a research psychologist and also a clinical psychologist. What I was watching was very similar to what I try to do in therapy, just through a different medium," she told me.

She described how she watched veterans—many of whom had never been in the ocean before—wade into the sea, become comfortable with the water around their feet, their hips, their shoulders, and eventually fully immerse themselves. The same change transpired atop a surfboard: dependent on physical ability, veterans first rode waves on their bellies, then on their knees, then on one leg and one knee, and eventually tried to stand and ride waves to shore.

"I witnessed this exposure element, and a sense of mastery as people were trying to reach a goal, succeed, and exceed their expectations and what they thought wasn't possible," she said.

She also witnessed the support the participants received from the community that was on the beach cheering them on: "Support you can't replicate in a group therapy setting."

Kristin said, "All of these things together led me to think surfing is therapeutic—what does the literature have to say?"

Motivated by her curiosity, she discovered Carly's study: *High-Intensity Sports for Posttraumatic Stress Disorder and Depression: Feasibility Study of Ocean Therapy With Veterans of Operation Enduring Freedom and Operation Iraqi Freedom*. But beyond that, she learned that there was very little literature on the effectiveness of surfing as a means of therapy at the time.

She soon joined the Naval Health Research Center and connected with Betty Michalewicz-Kragh, who had been seeing positive effects of surf therapy among service men and women for a few years and continued to explore this notion of surf therapy.

In the years that followed, Kristen helped author several ground-breaking studies that serve as the bedrock of literature for surf therapy's effectiveness on military personnel; today, Kristen is a Clinical Research Psychologist and Division Head of the Clinical Research Program at the Naval Health Research Center in San Diego. She also serves as the Principal Investigator on several Department of Defense-funded trials, where she conducts research on mental health treatments for service members.

"I come to surf therapy to assist the sector by being a clinical researcher," she said. She explained that when it comes to medical treatment, there are strict guidelines for what methodologies are acceptable, and she uses those guidelines to frame her research.

"I have focused on clinical outcomes, and on diagnosis. I use standardized assessments that are commonly used in the field, so we can actually compare results to psychotherapies, pharmacotherapies, and to other interventions," she said.

She did note that at the current time, it's important to think of surf therapy as "adjunctive care": most of the military personnel she studied over the last decade doing surf therapy were also participating in physical therapy, psychotherapy, and/or taking medications.

Amongst her other research, Kristen has focused on a singular question: "What does medical care look like when we add surf therapy, and how much benefit can we get from that?"

The studies she has conducted over the last decade provide a surprising answer.

Breaking the surface: Psychological outcomes among U.S. active duty service members following a surf therapy program examined the psychological outcomes of 74 active duty service members who were participating in the Naval Medical Center San Diego (NMCSD) surf therapy program. The studies' primary outcomes were published in

2019,[46] and they revealed that indeed, they were psychological benefits over the course of the six-week program, as well as during the 3–4 hour surf sessions—but scores on psychological measures rebounded by the start of the next session just one week later.

"This gave us an indication that having a surf session absolutely has psychological benefits," Kristen said. "But it doesn't last as long as a week."

Because of this, surf therapy isn't an elixir only to be experienced once; the study showed that to maintain therapeutic benefit, it must be done consistently—which therein lies a difficulty with those who don't live near the sea.

"Our recommendation is to try and have programs as often as feasible," Kristen said. "Betty [Michalewicz-Kraugh] will say it's like a medication dose that you need to take every day to get your benefit. The data seems to show that. The more frequent the therapy, the most advantageous it is for clinical benefit."

As a part of that study, Kristen and her team wanted to know how surfing's therapeutic properties differed by gender. In 2021, "*Gender Differences in Psychological Outcomes Following Surf Therapy Sessions among U.S. Service Members*" was published, and it found: "Women showed greater immediate improvements in depression/anxiety and positive affect compared with men-an important finding, given that surfing and military environments are often socially dominated by men."[47]

In "A randomized controlled trial of surf and hike therapy for U.S. active duty service members with major depressive disorder," Kristen sought to understand the effectiveness of outdoors therapy—specifically, hike and surf therapy—among 96 U.S. active duty service members with major depressive disorder (MDD).

Its findings, published in BMC Psychiatry in 2023, found "significant" and "clinically meaningful" improvements in depression severity as well as diagnosis for those who were participating in both Surf Therapy and Hike Therapy.

"The only difference between the groups was that Surf Therapy participants were more likely to lose their depression diagnosis at the 3-month follow-up," Kristen said.

The study's secondary outcomes (called "Psychological and functional outcomes following a randomized controlled trial of surf and hike therapy for U.S. service members") noted improvements in anxiety, psychological resilience, and social functioning amongst the collective group through the outdoors—and an even greater improvement for those who did surf therapy.

"Surf therapy may provide enhanced immediate effects on positive affect and pain," the study found.[48]

Kristen's goal has been to advance the surf therapy sector through clinical research, and it's obvious she's reached that goal—and, like a veteran who hasn't been in the ocean before but learns to stand and ride waves to shore—has exceeded that goal brilliantly. Looking forward, she's continuing to advocate for the sector the best way she knows how—by continuing to research.

"There are more surf therapy programs than surf therapy research programs," she told me. "Surf therapy research has the potential to have a great reach even beyond the local community"—she explained that because this research is open access, anyone with internet service can access it. "We really try and get our work out there so everyone who needs to use it and who would find it helpful can access it."

ℓℓℓ

With each step down the concrete walkway, the 820-foot USS Yorktown grows even bigger. Its stern sits on the left, with its bow on the right; behind it is the Arthur Ravenel Jr. Bridge, a massive two-pronged welcome beacon to Charleston, South Carolina.

Once inside the hangar of the former combat aircraft carrier, you're surrounded by historic planes that tell its story: the ship, commissioned in 1943, was renamed in honor of the previous Yorktown, which was sunk at the deadly Battle of Midway more than a year prior.

The Yorktown saw significant action as a battleship in World War II, and in the 1950s, it was updated to serve as an aircraft carrier in the Vietnam War.

Now, it acts as a floating history museum, a massive reminder of the effort and dedication it takes to defend freedom—and a place for those who fought to heal.

From the hangar, you follow the foot traffic to an elevator, which gets you onto the flight deck. Instead of seeing people walking the deck, marveling at its size, you see about 200 yoga mats spread across the rough coating on the historic deck with men and women—many of them current and former veterans in the United States Military—waiting for the class to begin.

The yoga class begins with everyone sitting in a comfortable position, and slowly moving into a downward dog, warming up the body. Warrior 1, Warrior 2, Warrior 3, and Tree Pose follow while the sun sinks towards the horizon, casting an orange glow over the scene.

Called Yoga on the Yorktown, it's far different from any yoga experience. This is because the yoga session is part of a surf therapy program that offers a different experience for veterans to heal from the traumas of war—with lifesaving results.

"I just knew I was going to die."[49]

This is how Andy Manzi described his two tours in Iraq as a Marine from 2003 to 2007, where he witnessed "intense firefights" and the death of other soldiers.

"Two weeks before I got home, we were engaged with the enemy. Just to go home and have to turn that off, I...felt like I had no control over myself. And I was afraid of myself."[50]

When Andy returned stateside, he carried no physical signs of injury. However, his brain told a different story. He continued to carry his experiences from the sands of Iraq with him every day, memories that he couldn't shake.

"One of the things I truly needed a few years after I got out was an opportunity to get out to do something different, to do something new to push myself again, and that's when I found surfing," he said.[51]

After buying a beat up surfboard at a yard sale and catching waves with the help of a friend, he was hooked. "Surfing changed my life and helped me to overcome those difficulties," he said.[52]

Andy knew that surfing could help other veterans, so, in 2015, he started Warrior Surf Foundation, which addresses post-service transition challenges such as PTSD, moral injury, survivor's guilt, and TBI through surf therapy, yoga, wellness sessions, and community.[53]

It was the start of an organization, but more so, the start of a journey of healing for hundreds of veterans.

ᕮᕮᕮ

Andy wasn't alone in his struggles after returning stateside. Yes, returning veterans, both combat and non-combat, can have obvious physical injuries; but it's what can't be seen that can be the most difficult injury of all.

The most talked about injury for returning veterans is Post Traumatic Stress Disorder (PTSD). With PTSD, as mentioned in Chapter 3, "time runs in the wrong direction, that is, from present back to the past."[54]

As far as a more clinical definition, the United States Department of Veteran Affairs defines it as a "mental health problem" that "can only develop after you go through or see a life-threatening event" and lists symptoms such as reliving the event, avoidance of what reminds you of the experience, and/or feeling on edge.

PTSD became an epidemic for returning veterans. Between 2000 and 2013 the number of claimants in the veteran's administration system receiving benefits for PTSD rose by almost 500 percent.[55] In addition, compensation seeking for this condition among veterans of the Iraq and Afghanistan wars is orders of magnitude greater than among veterans of previous wars.[56]

Another injury that can be obtained when deployed is called moral injury. By definition, moral injury occurs in response to acting or witnessing behaviors that go against an individual's values and moral beliefs.[57]

Stephanie Dasher, the Executive Director of Warrior Surf, communicated to me that her husband, Jordan, who spent 13 months in Iraq as a combat veteran, sees moral injury this way: "It's seeing people you trust take innocent lives, or being asked to do something outside of what not only your own upbringing tells is wrong, but that's also outside what the military has taught you is morally correct. It could even be following orders and firing rounds into what you thought was an empty building—only to find it was filled with women and children."

Jordan also explained that the military will create rules of engagement designed to keep everyone safe, and it's these rules that create space for discretionary judgment by military members who are under constant, adrenaline-fueled stress, which can open the door for moral injury—"Not just by the person who exercised judgment in a given situation, but by those soldiers around them," he said.

While there is an overlap with moral injury and PTSD, there are differences—including that moral injury can be more associated with suicide.

> *"One study found that perpetration-based events (events where someone perpetrated an act outside of one's values) were associated with more re-experiencing, guilt, and self-blame than were life threatening traumatic events. Reporting perpetration is also associated with greater suicidal ideation, even after adjusting for PTSD, depression, and substance use."*[58]

As Dave Grossman, a former Army Ranger, paratrooper, and psychology professor at West Point, puts it in *On Killing: The Psychological Cost of Learning to Kill in War and Society*: "It is the existence of the victim's pain and loss, echoing forever in the soul of the killer, that is at the heart of his pain."[59]

And that pain is moral injury.

Another mental health difficulty for returning soldiers is survivor's guilt, the haunting feelings of surviving an experience, such as surviving an IED explosion in Iraq, while others lost their lives. If a veteran follows the thought process *it should have been me killed in the explosion,* we're talking about survivor's guilt.

In *On Killing*, Dave Grossman, explains the dark psychology behind survivors' guilt—and why it can be so difficult to heal from.

> *"... The combat soldier appears to feel a deep sense of responsibility and accountability for what he sees around him. It is as though every enemy dead is a human being he has killed, and every friendly dead is a comrade for whom he was responsible.*

> *With every effort to reconcile these two responsibilities, more*
> *guilt is added to the horror that surrounds the soldier."*[60]

In addition to these injuries, veterans can return home with a traumatic brain injury (TBI), which can be caused by the impact of a nearby explosion, hitting your head inside a vehicle, or something striking you in the head. Symptoms can range from a headache to dizziness, difficulty concentrating or even becoming easily angered or frustrated.

For each of these cases, treatment centers around addressing PTSD. Overall, treatment is broken down between trauma-focused psycho-therapy with a counselor—Cognitive Processing Therapy (CPT), where you are taught skills to better understand how trauma affected your emotions; Prolonged Exposure (PE), where you literally repeat the experience over and over until it's no longer affecting you; Eye movement desensitization and reprocessing (EMDR) which helps alter the way you react to the memories of your trauma—and/or medication that is also used for depression.

According to the National Center for PTSD, 53 of 100 patients who receive one of these three therapies will no longer have PTSD. With medication alone, 42 of 100 will achieve remission.[61] While it's clear that these evidence based therapies are effective to some degree, they are still leaving a void of veterans looking for answers.

And that's the void Warrior Surf Foundation aims to fill.

ece

While every veteran's story for joining Warrior Surf Foundation is different, the reasons are the same: healing.

When Stephanie Dasher's husband, Jordan, returned from 13 months in Iraq as a combat veteran, he tried the prescribed therapy, but none of it worked. One of his therapists recommended Warrior Surf Foundation. For Stephanie, who loved the water, it was music to her ears. They arrived on the beach, met Andy Manzi, and similar to the other therapies, gave it a try.

"I saw my husband accept this challenge of surfing because he wasn't good at it right away," Stephanie told me. "Over time, I could see it was doing things for him."

She explained that instead of the Warrior Surf Foundation forcing a program on its participants, it's done the opposite and grown with its participants.

Initially, Warrior Surf focused on 6 surf sessions, and trauma therapy, which involved weekly group sessions you could attend.

"We found out quickly people don't want to do trauma therapy," Stephanie told me. "They don't want to do therapy actually, that's a scary word for a lot of people."

They also learned that 6 surf sessions weren't enough. They expanded the program to 12 weeks, and each veteran has certain tasks he or she needs to achieve to graduate. This includes 10 semi-private surf sessions, eight wellness coaching sessions, a 1:1 yoga session, and three group yoga sessions.

There are several reasons for this formula. Instead of giving participants just a few lessons, they want each participant to be a competent surfer, so he or she can get a dose of their surf therapy medicine on their own.

Much of their program takes place in community, and according to Stephanie, that's by design. "What we want to create is a community that is self-sustaining, where people have the tools to take care of themselves and in turn take care of other people. A lot of times we see people come into the program and are hesitant to make connections. So, by making the program a little bit longer, we're creating the opportunity for that connection to happen more organically."

The other piece of the puzzle is the eight wellness coaching sessions, led by a licensed social worker, along with licensed counselors. "We don't consider this therapy, we consider it positive psychology and psychoeducation," Stephanie told me. "You're getting a lot of tools you might get in therapy but you're learning to do it yourself. That's the ultimate goal of therapy is to parent your inner self."

The program is unique in that it combines so many elements, but that's strategic. "We know the brain becomes more malleable when it's in water," Stephanie said. "We know you have to be present in the moment. That's great then and there. But how do we take that experience and feeling and translate it back to our everyday lives?"

That's where yoga and wellness come into play.

"These are really powerful tools for mindfulness and psychoeducation, and we have surf wellness and yoga mirror each other," she said. "So when you go out and surf, you're going to take those tools you learned in wellness and apply them in surfing. That's a real life opportunity to practice something on a small level. So, if you get frustrated when you fall off a board, that's not a different kind of frustration than you might have in your day to day life. 'Ok I'm frustrated now, how do I respond in this moment here and how do I learn how to take that—using wellness coaching, using yoga for mindfulness—into my day to day life.' We want each piece of the program to feed each other, go in a circular motion of growth. We want to spiral up instead of spiral down."

In addition to this, they allow former participants to make an impact after graduation by serving as wellness coaches and mentors.

And the group yoga, of course, can involve Yoga on the Yorktown as well as yoga on the beach.

The results from the Warrior Surf Foundation's program speaks volumes. In 2022 alone, they have served more than 500 veterans and their family members, and conducted over 1,700 surf, wellness, and yoga sessions—with over 64 percent of participants receiving 6 or more wellness sessions (6 being considered a "therapeutic dose").

One graduate said it helped him create a life after the military:

"Before WSF, I was looking for integration, community building, and more importantly, I was actively seeking a relief valve

for all the accumulated stress that I have carried throughout my seventeen-year military career. The WSF family helped with all that from day one, not only did they provide me with all the tools I needed to defeat my stressors and fears to get back to society, but also introduced me with a way of life that increased dimensionality in my mental health and overall fitness. With their genuine interest in helping me with my challenges, the surf, wellness, and yoga, instructors crafted for me a path for a life after the military."[62]

One graduate said the program wants to help him improve not just in surfing, but in every aspect of his life.

"To be completely honest, surfing is actually pretty scary for me… When I was selected to attend the 12 week program, I had no idea if I would even make it through the first two hours. I told myself I wouldn't pass up this opportunity to force myself outside of my comfort zone, and the best way for me to deal with my issues is to face them head on—by challenging myself to do hard things. If it doesn't challenge you, it doesn't change you… Every time I walk into the ocean, I am actively challenging myself to face my fears by learning a skill and doing difficult tasks with people who sincerely want to see me win. Those people are the people who make me want to get better."

Today, the thriving Warrior Surf Foundation community collectively surf, collectively does yoga on the USS Yorktown, and collectively heals—an incredible result of one man buying a beat up surfboard at a garage sale and seeking to find unique ways to help his battle-torn mind.

An American flag—13 alternating red and white stripes and 50 white stars on a blue field—hangs on a pole, attached to a row of tents with the "Operation Surf" logo on them. The flag dances in the direction towards shore—an indication of the offshore winds, perfect for surfing.

Just south of the Avila Beach Pier, located in California's central coast, the Operation Surf event site is buzzing: green, yellow and blue surfboards line the sand, and now that the morning safety and instruction meeting is over, participants—wearing green rash guards on top of black O'Neill wetsuits—join the surf instructors—wearing red rash guards—and wade out to sea with a surfboard in tow.

Small waves roll through the break, and the surfing experience begins. Some with physical injuries ride on their belly; others attempt to stand and fall; others ride waves all the way to shore.

The entire day is dedicated to veterans healing from what it took to protect the American flag—a symbol of freedom, a symbol of justice— as it watches from above.

ᘓᘓᘓ

The VA and CDC has declared the rates of PTSD, suicide, and other injuries among military veterans as a National Health Crisis. An estimated 1 in 3 veterans are diagnosed with PTSD. Less than 40 percent seek help. 22 veterans commit suicide daily.[63]

Though it's impossible to quantify, what also factors into this is that soldiers are trained to not ask for help. They're trained to follow through with their orders, no matter what.

Operation Surf is on a mission to help this need, and it all started with Van Curaza.

Van forged his own path in surfing. After a professional career, he fell into a dangerous lifestyle of drugs and alcohol. After becoming sober, he founded a surf school called Van Curaza Surf School and a nonprofit called Amazing Surf Adventures. In addition to teaching the sport that he loved so much, he also helped at-risk youth.

Van had the opportunity to help a group of injured warriors in transition recovering from the Brooke Army Medical Center (BAMC) in San Antonio, Texas, to experience surfing. Seeing the magnitude of how it impacted them, he developed the curriculum for his new program Operation Surf based on his own perspective of his recovery and how it was parallel to helping veterans transition from the service into life back home.

Today, Operation Surf operates several programs, primarily in California's Central Coast, but also across the state and the country as well.

One of their programs is a week-long, all-inclusive surf program—which is at no cost to the veterans. Participants are welcomed by Operation Surf staff, volunteers and the local community at a beach-front hotel where they will spend their week together. The incredible week includes surfing, pre and post peer to peer support, daily yoga, mindfulness, group meals, nightly 'Recap Reel,' a closing award ceremony, and a paddle out to honor fallen heroes.

Operation Surf also runs a three month, locally focused program called OS3.0, where veterans commit to surf as a group at least twice a week.

In addition to these programs, they also have The Canteen, a virtual opportunity accessible to all current, past, and future participants that acts as a continual source of support and community.

Through each program, their goal is communicated through their motto: Changing lives one wave at a time.

Justin Martinez served for more than 20 years in the military, more specifically in the Army. He was part of the first wave of movement in the Iraq War after 9/11 and did a total of three tours of duty in the country. By the end of his tenure, he was a right hand man to the Commanding Officer of the Battalion.

Justin explained that when he left the service, he was given a folded up American flag, a printed thank you certificate from then-President Barack Obama. He attended a few transition briefs provided by the United States Veterans Affairs office, other resource channels, and that was it.

"When I got out, all that ended," Justin said.[64] "No one needed me. No one needed Chief Martinez anymore. I'm just Justin. I lost my identity."

Not only did Justin struggle with his identity—the connections and camaraderie he built throughout two decades in the military were gone.

In *On Killing*, Dave Grossman references a quote from Richard Gabriel, the author of *No More Heroes: Madness and Psychiatry in War*, on the topic of camaraderie within the military: "...in military writings on unit cohesion, one consistently finds the assertion that the bonds combat soldiers form with one another are stronger than the bonds most men have with their wives."[65]

A Vietnam veteran and ex-Rhodesian mercenary shared this sentiment, telling Dave:

> *"This is going to sound really strange, but there's a love relationship that is nurtured in combat because the man next to you—you're depending on him for the most important thing you have, your life, and if he lets you down, you're either maimed or killed. If you make a mistake the same thing happens to him, so the bond of trust has to be extremely close, and I'd say this bond is stronger than almost anything, with the exception of parent*

and child. It's a hell of a lot stronger than man and wife—your life is in his hands; you trust that person with the most valuable thing you have."[66]

"You get out and you don't have that connection and camaraderie with brothers and sisters in combat," Justin told me. "To me, that's something I was searching for."

In addition to this, Justin had a history of two traumatic brain injuries, one of which, a 3 millimeter spot on his brain had died. These symptoms, along with other injuries, led him to being on 10-15 pills of medication a day.

Struggling with all of it, in October of 2019, Justin went as far as putting a gun in his pocket and was on his way to commit suicide. His family members noticed his gun, and immediately called Justin's friend, a medic during the final deployment, to intervene. Had this not happened, it's likely he would have been another suicide statistic.

"At the time I felt no one understood the pain and depression I was enduring," Justin wrote. "I have suffered since and have fallen into a dark place which I continually battle, but since I have involved myself in organizations like Operation Surf, I feel like I'm a part of a team again. Van and his team have given me that purpose again and the ocean has healing elements that I cannot explain. The waves and ocean are definitely my zen and the entire staff that operation surf is what drives me towards internal healing so that I can be an advocate and example of what operation surf does for the veterans it serves."

Today, Justin is the program manager, is responsible for all programs within the organization and a mentor to those on Avila Beach and the site of other surf events. "Surfing is my medication," he said. "At

Operation Surf we're given opportunities to heal properly—without medications."

Justin isn't the only one who has been tremendously impacted by Operation Surf. The Netflix documentary *Resurface* chronicles the story of other veterans, including Bobby, an Iraq War Veteran.

Bobby had severe PTSD, which manifested at home, in the car, and was taking too many medications to count. But none of it was helping. Operation Surf had a slot open for him to participate, and he was going to go—but, in his mind, it was going to be the last thing he would do.

"I was gonna go surfing, go home, make sure everything was in order, and I was going to get my gun and commit suicide," Bobby said.[67]

But the connections he made—and the effect surfing had—made him change his plans.

> *"When I caught that wave, it felt like a part of me died. The Bobby going through life, so much pain and guilt, that guy died out there that day. And I could feel the ocean's heartbeat as if it was this living, breathing thing. It wasn't death and destruction and trauma and hell. I close my eyes to go sleep and the only thing I could think about was catching that next wave. I'm not saying the first wave cured me. But the ocean is the one place I know I can go to for peace."[68]*

Along with these powerful testimonials, I discovered that Operation Surf has incredible data to share on the program's efficacy.

"The Impact of Ocean Therapy on Veterans with Posttraumatic Stress Disorder," authored by Dr. Russell Crawford, a Licensed Professional Counselor and military veteran, revealed that participants with Operation Surf experienced:

- 36 percent decrease in PTSD symptoms
- 47 percent decrease in depression
- 68 percent increase in self-efficacy[69]

The study highlighted a significant reduction in depression symptoms, as measured by the BDI-II score, for combat veterans immediately after ocean therapy and at the 30-day time point.[70]

The study also found there was a correlation between the population of veterans seeking an adrenaline rush, and finding it with surfing: "Veterans with PTSD frequently seek experiences and activities that provide an adrenaline rush."[71]

> *"Research and this study support that ocean therapy can be a substitute for illegal adrenaline oriented behaviors, as well as extreme aggressive and physical behaviors at various intervals in the life of these patients. Surfing like other extreme sports, produces an adrenaline rush and suggests that programs designed with this type of group activity can be highly affective and can be introduced when needed to relieve PTSD symptoms and increase self-efficacy, as well as reduce depression."[72]*

Along with this, Dr. Crawford did discover that, just as Justin alluded to by saying "surfing is my medicine," there is some science there.

"Harnessing the power of the need for adrenaline exhibited by many veterans, without the use of medications, has huge appeal to sustaining the quality of life for the veteran and their family."[73]

Another fascinating study on Operation Surf and this notion of surf therapy for veterans was conducted by Dr. Jon Ossie and the University of San Diego in partnership with Whoop. Using Whoop—a wearable tracker that monitors your heart rate, sleeping patterns and more—he was able to study Operation Surf participants like never before.

He found:

- REM minimum sleep in all participants increased 47 percent. "Rapid Eye Movement (REM) sleep is associated with the consolidation of emotional memory and has been suggested to be the stage of sleep during which emotion is regulated. This is when the brain dreams, processes information, and stores memories."[74]
- 82 percent of participants saw an increase in their Heart Rate Variability (HRV) mean for the 30 days after the event compared to the event. "Higher HRV for greater variability between heart beats indicates that the body has a strong ability to tolerate stress or is strongly recovering from prior accumulated stress.[75]
- 65 percent of participants saw their HRV median increase 30 days after the event compared to before the event. [76]

This data and countless testimonials show that Operation Surf is meeting the need—a need deemed National Health Crisis—one veteran at a time and one wave at a time.[77]

ᗕᗕᗕ

From Folly Beach, South Carolina to Avila Beach, California and many places in between, it's inspiring to see how organizations, using surfing, are helping to heal the traumas created through war. But they aren't just surfing.

Building off the data pioneered by the likes of Carly Rogers, Betty Michalewicz-Kragh and Kristen Walter, practitioners and organizations are continuing to collect data to further prove surf therapy's efficacy—with the hopes of it being more available in the years to come.

Above all, they're creating a new way—driven by evidence—for us to view mental health among service members.

3

INNER CITIES, TOWNSHIPS & RADIATION ZONES: SURF THERAPY FOR AT-RISK YOUTH

I t's 9:30am in Masiphumelele—also known as Masi—a township located outside of Cape Town in South Africa. Forty to 50 children and young adults line the pavement as the fabled Table Mountain looms in the background.

Some are sitting, others are standing. All are waiting.

The scars of the apartheid—a racial segregation movement that forced non-white South Africans to move into specific districts, also known as townships—are in clear view. Living areas are smashed together, some of which are nothing more than shipping crates. Sounds of violence fill the air, but sirens don't follow the noise.

A beat up Toyota truck, with surfboards tied to its roof, comes into view. The group of youth become visibly excited; some who have already experienced this before look to be the most jubilant; others who have only heard about it look on with curious eyes.

Inside the truck is a driver, an Englishman named Tim Conibear, and a passenger, Apish Tshetsha, who is a native to South Africa.

They both open the truck's creaky doors and help the children into the extended bed of the truck, which can fit quite a number of those waiting. They promise they'll be back for the rest soon.

With everyone loaded, they begin their trek to Muizenberg Beach, a few kilometers away. They arrive at the beach and the surfing soon commences. Watching the scene, it looks like a group of kids going surfing. But it's far more than that.

Although they didn't realize it, taking kids from Masiphumelele to the ocean was the first step of a movement.

A movement that would see thousands of children, who all had tremendous trauma exposure and chronic toxic stress, experience relief.

A movement that would create jobs for hundreds of South Africans who call the townships home.

And a movement that would reshape and redefine how the South African community would view mental health.

ℯℯℯ

Tim Conibear had ventured from his native England to South Africa for passion, and to fund his adventure, he worked for a surf tour guide company.

Instead of spending his time in the country's tourist attractions, he wanted to see what he called "the real flavor of South Africa," and that was located in the four townships that surround Cape Town.

"The image I had been encouraged to have of townships was dangerous and unwelcoming," Tim told me. "You didn't tend to see people like me going into a township. But it was actually the opposite."

Tim explained how a vibrant culture lined the streets of Masi; music on every corner, the smells of a family BBQ, the clicks that followed the native tongue of Xhosa; a strong sense of community.

In his time in the townships, Tim learned of the challenges that the population faced, and he wanted to help. The only problem was that not many Englishmen had done a lot of good in South Africa before.

He made a friend playing football named Apish, a fixture in the local community, and together they decided to take kids and young adults surfing in Muizenberg Beach, Cape Town.

Tim and Apish put the word out that on an upcoming Saturday morning, around 9am, they would stop in Masi and take anyone who wanted to the beach and surf.

On that day, they arrived to find three or four kids waiting on the pavement. They took them to the beach and gave them surf lessons. Afterwards, they got them some food and dropped them back off in Masi.

The next week, Tim wondered if the same number would be waiting. When he arrived, he was surprised to see about 15 kids on the pavement. In the small vehicle he and Apish were using, it was clear that Tim would have to make several trips while Apish led the surf instruction.

The following week, as Tim and Apish drove into Masi, they wondered if there would be the same number of kids, or less. When they arrived, they were shocked to see 45 to 50 people waiting for him—and that's when they realized they were going to need a bigger vehicle.

Using relationships from his tour company job, Tim inquired if there were any vehicles he could utilize for this rapidly-growing surf experience. He was given a truck with an extra-long bed that had been run into the ground.

"It was the cheapest of the cheap," Tim remembers. "The front bench in the cab was rusted, and I couldn't move it forward or backwards. I'm quite tall, so my knees were around my ears."

In addition to this, the steering column was rusted, and it couldn't go faster than 30 KMH, but Tim said that "its enormous flatbed could fit 20 or 30 people."

The truck filled the need, and donated wetsuits and surfboards helped fill other needs.

The surf club was widely successful—and Tim, who considers himself "infuriatingly curious and inquisitive,"[78] wanted to know why.

Tim and Apish decided to ask the participants as they drove to the beach and during surf lessons: *why do you keep coming with us to surf? Why do you wait on the pavement as early as 7am for us to pick you up around 9 or 9:30am?*

They received answers they expected—surfing was exciting; it was a way to see something outside of the township where they lived. But there was one answer that they didn't anticipate hearing: "we can talk, and people listen to us."[79]

It floored them: some kids had been waiting on the pavement since as early as 7am—waiting two hours just to be listened to.[80]

When Tim heard this, he wanted to know why the participants weren't being listened to. He wanted to learn what it was like to be a child in Masi.

"My impressions were that, yes, it's a difficult place but it also seemed vibrant and a place I'd like to live," Tim said. "There was something about the community I didn't understand yet."

With the help of Elizabeth Benninger, who studied psychology and children's well-being at the University of the Western Cape, Tim was able to understand that children living in townships go through tremendous stress and trauma.

The data at the time said that youth located in the area go through up to eight traumatic events on an annual basis. These "traumatic events" could be anything from sexual abuse to physical abuse, the incarceration of a parent, or the death of a family member. On the contrary, Tim might go through a few—in a lifetime.

"The stat we found at the time was that, in Masi, 60,000 people lived, there was no police station, no fire service, two social workers, one primary school, and one high school," Tim said.

In addition to this, there was 60 percent unemployment, and most families were surviving on a child grant, which provided 300 rand, equivalent to $30 a month.

"This is why kids are waiting on the side of the road to have a conversation," he said.[81]

Tim, who sought therapy for a traumatic experience prior to venturing to South Africa, began to think about how intimidating sitting with a counselor was, and how in the silence, you attempt to fill it with conversation. And how surf therapy was such a different experience—a much more welcoming and fun one.

"We found that surfing was the medium to have that conversation," he said. "We found when you move that to the beach, silence doesn't matter because you can catch a wave. You can pick up conversations when you want to. Surfing breeds confidence, creates social connections, naturally conversation strikes up. Surfing is a non-threatening way to open conversations with kids who would struggle to have those conversations in their day to day life."

He continued: "It all came from that first realization that the kids don't come just to surf, they come for something a lot more."

"I realized this is more than surfing," said Apish. "I can really have an impact on young peoples' lives…Caring, being consistent, showing up, listening to what they're going through and helping them feel safe. I didn't have space like that growing up. I guess that's why I wanted to do it for them."[82]

Instead of just taking the population surfing, Tim and Apish wanted to take the next step and create a safe space at the beach where the kids could share their struggles. Tim imagined that was something they could train people to do. In addition, he looked at Apish, and given the high rate of unemployment in the area, thought this could

be a way for the adults in the area to have a job. And maybe the organization, Tim thought, could support people like Apish just as much
as it supports the participants.

Waves for Change, founded in 2011, was born.

ᘒᘒᘒ

More than a decade after Tim and Apish were picking up children in a
beat up truck, the organization continues to address the mental health
need for a large at-risk young adult population.

Similar to Tim, I wanted to learn what it's like to be a child in
current day Masi. And what I found was startling.

Elizabeth Benninger conducted a study that examined how children within urban communities in Cape Town "construct and assign
meaning to the 'self.'" Published in 2016, it found:

> *"The discussions around their feelings revealed an underlying
> sense of helplessness and vulnerability, which they associated
> with their identity as children. The streets within the partic-
> ipants' neighborhoods were characterized by violence with
> limited spaces of safety. These safe spaces could only be accessed
> through 'dodging bullets, cars, and gangsters.'"[83]*

The same study showed just how much these instances—"dodging
bullets, cars and gangsters"—affected the children in their most formative years."

> *"Male Participant 1: There was a kidnapping, this has affected
> us a lot because the kid who was kidnapped had his body cut
> up, put in a black bag, and buried ... This spreads a lot of fear
> amongst the kids.*

Male Participant 2: There was also a poison and a lot of kids died because a man poisoned children in the community, this makes it scary to be a child."[84]

If the streets and surrounding community aren't safe, the only option for children to find safety is in their living quarters. But Benninger discovered that, in many cases, wasn't safe either:

"The housing infrastructure in the participants' communities consisted of high density and overcrowded apartments or shacks, where there were limited spaces for play. The children evocatively referred to being "imprisoned" in their homes, which forced them to forfeit an important aspect of their child identity; the ability to play safely outside."[85]

More recently, in 2022, Waves for Change conducted a study to see how many children were affected by violence.

"All 233 participants in the study endorsed extremely high rates of exposure to violence, such that 100 percent of participants had witnessed violence, and all but two participants (98.2 percent) had directly experienced violence."[86]

I asked Tim if the mental services had improved since his original examination of the population and their needs. He said that mental services do exist, but "they're only at the tip of the pyramid."

He continued: "When you're living on 30 rand a day with no health insurance in a community where mental health isn't spoken about, you don't think to ask for help," he said. "For the population we work with, there is no word for depression in Xhosa and mental health isn't a term widely used in these communities."

Another examination by the organization found the devastating combination of abuse and, similar to a decade ago, few mental health services.

> "...the same demographic that is disproportionately exposed to abuse, crime and violence is that which has the least access to mental healthcare services and an even slimmer chance of being attended to by a psychologist who looks like them and speaks their language."[87]

Therein lies the treatment gap, and where Waves for Change, acting as an early prevention tool, exists to fill the void.

In their model, children who need intervention are identified and supported. This leads to less children needing expensive treatment and becoming ill, reducing the burden on the mental health system.

For each individual, the Waves for Change program begins when he or she is referred by schools, social workers, local clinics or other community partners.

After that, the individual attends weekly surf sessions, lasting two hours, for 10 months. They are supervised by Waves for Change coaches, ages 18-25 who are trained in what's called "the five pillar method."

The five pillars are:

- Connection to consistent mentor support and a positive peer group
- Access to a safe space
- Access to fun and challenging new tasks
- Practicing social and emotional skills
- Connection to new opportunities and support systems[88]

In addition, the coaches are supervised by psychologists, and it's these psychologists who lead group sessions with up to 60 children at a time.[89]

I was curious to see what data they had. The five pillar model— utilizing surf therapy—has yielded the following results:

- 96 percent of participants reported feeling happier
- 93 percent of participants reported feeling more confident
- 94 percent of participants were better able to calm down when they feel sad, angry or scared
- 79 percent of participants have improved heart visibility rate
- "Our service reduces the risk of mental health challenges escalating during adolescence/adulthood, and reduces burden on the MH system in vulnerable communities."[90]

Another study confirmed that the Waves for Change's Surf Therapy program is an efficacious, trauma-informed intervention for violence-exposed children and youth.[91]

While those studies provided a solid base of evidence, I found one of their more recent studies the most fascinating. The goal was to measure how toxic stress affected the participants, and how the program, which included surfing, could help that.

It starts with understanding what toxic stress actually is. "Toxic stress is a buildup of cortisol, adrenaline and stress," Tim told me. "They are your body's natural response, but if it's happening all the time, that build-up becomes toxic and changes the way your body functions."

This causes a toxic stress response, "which can lead to lifelong problems in learning, behavior, and physical and mental health."[92] More specifically, this can lead to headaches, increased heart rate, changes in appetite, which can affect weight and much more.

The next question was how to measure toxic stress. Tim and the organization worked with Dr. Wendy D'Andrea of the New School

University in New York and the global Laureus Sport for Good Foundation, using Heart Rate Variability (HRV) as a measure.

> *"HRV is simply a measure of the variation in time between each heartbeat; and is controlled by the autonomic nervous system (ANS); which is divided into the sympathetic and the parasympathetic nervous system (SNS and PNS). While some SNS activity is needed for attention, big increases in SNS activity lead to a state of fight or flight. Increases in PNS lead to relaxation, self-awareness, attention, and connection, however, too much can lead to shutting down under stress."[93]*

Waves For Change children would see "at least" eight traumatic experiences per year—compared to children in the USA who would experience five in their entire childhood.[94]

That toxic stress negatively affects the hippocampus, prefrontal cortex, and amygdala. The results of this are expansive: it can affect decision making, self-regulation, fear processing, memory, and stress management, along with mental health problems such as behavioral disorders, suicidality, and anxiety.[95]

The lower the HRV, the more the individual is over-responding, is unhealthy, and has an imbalance in the heart and mind. The higher HRV, the more the individual has a greater sense of wellbeing, is relaxed, and has a low risk of high blood pressure.

These were measured over the course of a 10 week surf therapy program. And, in the end, "Positive program effects seem to occur after eight weeks and are sustained thereafter."[96]

More specifically, the study found the following among participants:

- Improvements in HRV
- Improved self-esteem

- Reduced impulsivity
- Improved attention (less inattention)
- Increased closeness to others
- *More* stress, which, given the extremely low stress reporting at baseline, suggests an increase in accuracy in self-report data, as the intervention was implemented.

"After eight sessions, you see the autonomic nervous system begin to change and regulate," Tim told me. "Using surf therapy, we were teaching kids how to self soothe and feel calmer and addressing the underlying issue of toxic stress."

What is impressive about both Wave for Change's story and data is that it hasn't been a flash-in-the-pan trend—it's been a sustainable organization that has become an integral helping hand for the surrounding communities.

As of 2022, over 8,500 kids have experienced surf therapy through Waves for Change.[97] In addition to this, each year, Waves for Change trains 45 coaches how to be a caring adult. The goal was for the organization to exist for coaches as well—and it's been coming to fruition.

The ultimate example of the process working is a participant becoming a volunteer or coach, and that's happened with many individuals in the program. One Waves for Change coach said:

> "…I was born in Cape Town and currently live in Lavender Hill. I got involved with W4C at the age of 12 years old as a participant. After I matriculated, I got the opportunity to become a Junior Coach for two years, becoming a Senior Coach in 2022. W4C has had an impact on my life since the age of 12 by creating a safe space for me. I had a caring adult mentor who was always there to check-in on me and my feelings. W4C provided me with both the life skills and life lessons needed to help me think more positively, to have a positive attitude and positive thoughts and a better understanding of what mental health

is. I am now a caring adult who is trying to make a positive change in other children's lives. I am a role model and mentor to the kids in our programme. I love working with every single child and being able to witness the change within them.[98]

Helping participants, helping coaches, curating data…What's also impressive about Waves for Change is that their model has expanded to help train and create autonomous surf therapy organizations in countries around the world where mental health services are "under resourced."[99]

As of 2023, there are 12, including Senegal, Sierra Leone, Somalia, Kenya, Peru, Trinidad and Tabago, and more.

This expansion led to more surf therapy—and more data. Authored by Dr. Jamie Marshall, one study found one child participant in post-war torn Liberia say, "I feel happy when I surf because it takes stress from my mind."[100]

In another location, Sierra Leone, Jamie found "in this uncontrolled study, three out of four surf therapy sites analyzed were associated with significant large positive effects on participant well-being."[101]

"It goes back to the initial experiences in Masi, recognizing people who can make a change in the community themselves," Tim told me. "It wasn't us bringing people in and running our own program…it was 'let's help you start this for your community.'"

Tim explained how in the early days, he became a driver and went to surf shops trying to get gear while Apish took the lead on the beach. "Quite often, there's a temptation to be the person delivering it and at the forefront. As an organization, we've been lucky to have this mentorship concept of servant leadership. If it's going to last, if it's going to be sustainable in 20 or 30 years, the community has to lead it. They offer training, help them with gear and evaluation so they can impact and write up reports, and take it to donors and get funding with the goal of being an autonomous organization."

And that's exactly what has happened—Waves for Change has stood the test of time, helping bridge the gap of mental health services in South Africa, while providing jobs for locals and cultivating a generation who understands the importance of mental health.

ⓔ ⓔ ⓔ

It's a chilly morning on Rossnowlagh Beach, a massive expanse where the sea meets rolling green hills of Northern Ireland.

Surf instructors with blue rash guards that read "Liquid Therapy" are interacting with about 20 teenagers on the sand that's so compact you can park a car on it. The first thing you notice is that these interactions are coming from hand signals, not words; upon closer inspection, the surf instructors are speaking English, while the participants are speaking Russian and Belarussian.

When you ask why the language barrier exists, the reply from Tom Losey, the Founder of Liquid Therapy is shocking. His response also shows that while this looks like just a surf session—a group getting together to learn how to ride waves in the sea—it's far more than that.

The young participants are visiting from what's referred to as "most toxic landscape in the world,"[102] Chernobyl and the surrounding area of Belarus. According to Tom, they're getting in the water to surf, yes. But on this day, they'll also be cleansing from the effects of one of the worst man-made disasters in human history.

ⓔ ⓔ ⓔ

After managing a surf school in Ireland and taking children with special needs surfing for years, Tom Losey saw the need for a surf therapy program in Ireland. Liquid Therapy, which began in 2011, exists to be a gateway to the ocean for "anyone who struggles or cannot participate in a mainstream environment."

The organization has nine different programs, including working with those struggling with negative mental health, physical challenges, trauma, autism and more, all on a 1:1 basis. One of those programs takes children from Chernobyl and the surrounding Belarus region surfing.

On the morning of April 26, 1986, no one could fathom that the day would see one of the most dangerous man-made events in history and have reverberating effects in the generations to come. At the nuclear power plant in Chernobyl, Number Four RBMK reactor melted down—a terrifying combination of human error and a deeply flawed design. A subsequent explosion blew the roof off the reactor, which blasted invisible radioactive particles skyward—"The Chernobyl explosion put 400 times more radioactive material into the Earth's atmosphere than the atomic bomb dropped on Hiroshima."[103]

The radiation then fell on the land, injecting radioactivity into the ecosystem and food chain, and in the process, the surrounding population.

Today, Pripyat, the city the nuclear power plant is located in, remains closed off and uninhabited—and some scientists estimate it won't return to normal for at least 3,000 years.[104]

But a large population still lives near the radioactive area. One of the many reasons is the inability to move financially. For those in the neighboring country of Belarus, which is just six miles from the site of the meltdown, 70 percent of the fallout from the Chernobyl accident landed there, contaminating 23 percent of the country to a level of over one curie per square kilometer.[105]

This disaster set off a socioeconomic bomb too; because the surrounding areas remain radioactive, businesses, jobs, and a livable income are hard to come by.

"There's no infrastructure, no investment, no opportunity," Tom told me. "You see the families are desperate for their kid to get out."

That's where Liquid Therapy comes in.

"Here in Ireland, we have a strong community of organizations and charities that provide respite from children from Chernobyl," Tom said.

He became aware of a large program that allowed children and young adults to be hosted by families in Ireland—"over the past 30 years, 25,500 children from Belarus and western Russia have visited Ireland as part of the annual summer rest and recuperation programme."[106]

It's a program that Dr. Easkey Britton, a pro Irish surfer, scientist, and surf therapy advocate, saw firsthand when she was a young girl.

> *"The Chernobyl nuclear disaster happened the same year I was born and I met some of the kids who came to Donegal for respite and health restoration, same age as me, thin and pale as ghosts, many recovering from cancer treatment (or still suffering from it), others terminally ill despite their youth, and they had never even seen the sea. That blew my little mind. I'll always remember the impact on them of being in the sea for the first time when they came to my local beach at Rossnowlagh for a day. Looking back, it was a moment that firmly cemented my belief in the power of the sea to heal, to connect across language barriers, across cultures and the power of play. Just the simple joy of it all and how it transformed, even if only momentarily, their emotional and physical wellbeing, their sense of awe and wonder, experiencing themselves in this fluid, animated world so full of life and energy, in a new way."[107]*

"I have been in the Chernobyl Children Appeal for eleven years and have hosted children from Ukraine & Belarus for ten years," said Eveline Smith, who serves as a host to the population in need. "The children that come are mostly from the country and away from the city areas, they come from very basic families for whom every day is a struggle to work and earn some money to survive."

The program takes young teenagers on adventures, such as visiting animal parks, caves, barbecues or going to a waterpark…"opportunities they don't get at home," Tom says.

It was obvious for Tom, a man with surfing always on his mind, to take them surfing through Liquid Therapy.

At each event, usually held at Rossnowlagh Beach, there are roughly 20 participants who have never been to the beach, never seen the ocean, let alone surfed before, who are trusting strangers who don't speak their language.

Despite these obstacles, after a visually-led beach instruction, they join Liquid Therapy's surf instructors with a surfboard and wade into the sea where they learn the international language of surfing.

"Once they're in the water, there's no conversation," Tom told me. "There's thumbs up, shakas, high fives…surfing transcends so many barriers, including language."

Tom spoke about how surfing can be therapeutic mentally, from boosting their confidence to facing adversity and being forced to focus on the present, not the challenges that await them when they return home. What I found most shocking was that surfing, and the adventure program as a whole, has tremendous physical benefits.

"Every month a child spends outside that zone in Chernobyl, their life expectancy goes up six months," Tom told me, explaining that the combination of clean air and saline in the water helps flush their systems in a beneficial way.

"Research has shown that the children, who come from impoverished backgrounds and state-run institutions, get a health reprieve from the toxic environment and high levels of radiation to which they have been exposed. Their radiation levels drop by nearly 50 percent during their month-long stay."[108]

Plus, the data says there's not just short term benefits, but long term benefits as well.

"Doctors in Belarus say that a four week holiday boosts the children's immune systems for at least two years, helping them to resist, or recover from, serious illness."[109]

Facing adversity, focusing on the present, cleansing…At the end of the day, what's most important to the participants, is that this type of therapy, compared to other forms, is fun. "None of them wanted to leave [the beach] when it was over," Eveline told me.

ꙅꙅꙅ

A white passenger van makes several stops throughout San Francisco's lower-income neighborhoods so early in the morning that the street-lights are still lit.

Yellow, pink and blue foam surfboards are tied to its roof, and a bumper sticker on the back of the van reads "MeWater Foundation," written around a crashing wave.

Apartment after apartment, Eddie Donnellan and Tim Gras—white males in their 50s—knock on doors on the chilly morning. Teenagers of color, with sleepy faces, pile into the van until nearly every seat is filled.

With everyone on board, the surf adventure begins. But the van turns the opposite direction of the chilly Pacific surrounding San Francisco; instead, it heads inland on Interstate 5 South.

Some of the passengers doze off; others stare at the scenery out the windows: the rising sun lights up empty fields and fall-colored mountains. Instead of the smell of a salty sea, the unpleasant smell of cows, chickens and farmland fills the van.

After more than a three-hour trek, the van turns off of the interstate, and minutes later, it stops in front of a massive gate that reads "SURF RANCH." The gate, as if from the Willy Wonka Chocolate Factory, opens and welcomes the group to the surf experience of a lifetime.

Inside is one massive rectangular pool with what looks to be a train stretching from end to end directly in the middle. Calm and glassy water greets everyone's eyes, but with a flick of a switch, it transforms into the world's most perfect wave, created by 11-time World Champion Kelly Slater.

With anticipation at its peak, nothing can happen fast enough for the participants: the boards can't come off the van soon enough, the wetsuits can't be put on quickly enough.

Soon, the group is sitting in the shallower end of the wave pool: Eddie and Tim have participants on surfboards, while others will paddle themselves. The switch is flipped, and a perfect wave pushes through, a scene that will make every surfer go mad with jealousy.

As the wave reaches the group, it turns into whitewash. Shouts reverberate, and seconds later, participants are up and riding. It's an extraordinary scene. But it's even more extraordinary when you realize what it took for this to happen—and the stories just beneath the surface.

Being invited to surf at Kelly Slater's Surf Ranch is, well, a fantasy. The only way to receive the "golden ticket" is if you know Kelly himself. Or, in the rare chance you know the crew who helps run and operate the Surf Ranch, you could receive entry then.

The only other way to enter its famed doors is by paying, which is an exorbitant cost—daily rentals can range from $50,000-$70,000.[110] Most surfers today know they'll likely never surf it or even see it in person. It will always be a fantasy hidden by the mist of exclusivity in the farmland of California.

When Eddie and Tim, two lifelong surfers, received the golden ticket for entry, they could have taken it for themselves. Instead, they brought participants from MeWater, the surf therapy Foundation they started.

In one of the most exclusive and expensive surfing locations in the world, teenagers of color were having the time of their lives. Had Eddie and Tim not helped and mentored them through MeWater, these participants could have been in a far different situation—trapped in a bad lifestyle, imprisoned, or even worse, dead.

ᘓᘓᘓ

At the 2019 International Surf Therapy Conference, I spoke on a panel about how surfing can help populations in need, drawing on stories from my first book, *Waves of Healing*.

Sitting in front of a few hundred people in person and online, I expected to talk, but I wasn't expecting to listen.

Eddie and Tim were on the panel alongside me, and on the stage, I couldn't believe the story I was hearing—not only did Eddie and Tim give their golden ticket to the MeWater participants; without MeWater, the population they serve could instead be trapped in a deadly lifestyle. On top of that, many MeWater participants have had negative experiences with white men, yet Eddie and Tim, two white males, were acting as their mentors.

After the panel, I couldn't help but ask Eddie more questions. What followed was multiple conversations on selflessness, the impact of mentorship, and surf therapy.

Nearly a million people inside a 50-square mile area make up the melting pot that is San Francisco. Because the city is surrounded by three coasts, and because you can see water from so many vantage points throughout the city, you'd think the ocean would be a significant part of the culture.

"Even though the Bay is a mile away, mother nature for the majority of these kids doesn't exist," Eddie told me. "It's a cement world."

There are color barriers, trust barriers, and race barriers that, at the end of the day, prevent those from low income neighborhoods getting to the ocean.

In these low income neighborhoods, the choice of doing what is right versus what is easy is blurred. First responder sirens, the noise of trauma, violence, drug abuse, incarceration, are like a broken record that won't stop repeating. And within these neighborhoods are impressionable teenagers and young adults.

A recent study found just how large the low-income population in San Francisco is:

"Black and Latino residents are overrepresented among the region's very low income and low-income families. Black

and Latino residents make up 46 percent of very-low income
families but just 13 percent of high-income families. White
residents, on the other hand, comprise just a quarter of very
low-income families but 54 percent of high-income families,
even though they make up 40 percent of the region's overall
population."[111]

"There's a lot of uncertainty and not clear safety if you step out of the door in these neighborhoods," Eddie told me. "Going down the wrong path is not hard. There's not a lot of opportunity for these kids."

"These are kids who have had disrupted upbringings," said Niki Berkowtiz, a Clinician and Clinical Supervisor.[112] "They live in really poor neighborhoods, they are exposed to a lot of trauma that comes from parents being incarcerated, drug use, a lot of community violence. That impacts a lot of the kid's behavior and moods…"

For nearly 20 years, Eddie and Tim worked together at the Edgewood Center for Children and Families, a residential treatment center, which has a history of working with some of the most challenging children and young adults in the state. Eddie and Tim's focus was "trauma informed care" and running outdoor summer camps. Eddie notes that while he's not a licensed therapist, he has decades of direct care experience, along with managing and directing programs.

For two lifelong and passionate surfers, making the bridge from programs at Edgewood and outdoor summer camps to taking the participants surfing was obvious, and when they saw firsthand the therapeutic effects surfing had, they founded MeWater.

MeWater's mission is to "provide day and overnight surf camps to youth, families, and groups, with a mental health approach to mindfulness, empowerment, and exposure to the ocean and the great outdoors." Their population is 90 percent children of color.

On the morning of a typical MeWater surf day, you can find Eddie driving throughout the low income neighborhoods in the MeWater passenger van, surfboards likely tied to the roof, and picking up participants who had signed up ahead of time or have a history with the foundation.

"You have to be aware of the dynamics of the neighborhood," Eddie told me. "If I knock on someone's door and the participant isn't there, I've learned to not ask questions or not tell them they were supposed to come surf… I thank them and tell them we'd love to take them surfing next time."

Eddie and a handful of participants meet others at a nearby beach. This can range from other participants to surf instructors, and often, MeWater has a nurse, psychiatrist, or therapist on the beach as well.

Once wetsuits are on—which is one of the more difficult aspects—Eddie will have everyone sit in a circle and introduce themselves. Then, he'll give a safety talk that acts as a metaphor for what MeWater does.

After explaining that the participants will be in the shallow area and don't have to fear drowning, he says, "We're going to help you when you fall down. Because if you do, one of us will be there to help you up."

Eddie told me: "It is really important to me that we are helping to build a trust-based connection that goes much further than just in the water."

After safety instruction, Eddie explains that there's no expectations for the day. If participants want to surf, they'll have the chance to. If participants want to build sandcastles, they can do that as well.

"There's no structure, and it's by design," Eddie tells me. "Everything is their choice." Even when they break for lunch, many participants won't want to get out of the water, so, along with the surf instructors, they'll eat as they keep surfing.

It may look like a single surf event. But it's days like this that have changed the lives of several of MeWater's participants, like Anthony.

Anthony's grandmother, Shirley, took him in when he was six months old. He doesn't know where his mother is to date. Shirley explains the circumstances of his father, "big Anthony." She explained that after an altercation between his mother and his father, his mother called the police.

"…And they took him. While he was there [in prison], he had an asthma attack and they didn't go see about him. And that's where he passed. In a cell on the floor by himself. And that's what happened to big Anthony."[113]

Anthony Junior became a staple in the MeWater surf program, bouncing his grades, questions to Eddie as he grew older. He became a volunteer, then an intern, and today attends college at San Francisco State University.

"Surfing makes me feel calmer," he said.[114] "I get angry at life sometimes, but I always feel better when I get in the ocean."[115]

MeWater also changed the life of Ollis. Raised in group homes with no parents or family, he found a family with MeWater, and found surfing therapeutic. "I feel like the water humbled me and changed the way I thought about things," he told me. "It made me more mature, more calm. I feel like I can actually feel emotions better and understand why I can feel them [when I'm in the water]. I can feel at ease."

Beyond that, Ollis found the community and mentorship lifesaving.

"If [MeWater] wasn't in my life, being in the environment I grew up in…I would find myself in a darker lifestyle," he told me. "I feel like I would gravitate to using drugs and being in the street."

These testimonials point to what Eddie and MeWater value above all: mentorship. So how does Eddie, a white male in his 40s, mentor teenagers and young adults growing up in low income areas?

I asked Eddie about his comment in a recent interview with Patagonia where he said, "When some of the kids show up, you can tell that they haven't had many positive experiences with white people."[116]

"As a white male, I feel like it's important that I say that," Eddie told me. "I have a responsibility as a white male to call things as I see them and hear what's being said back."

For Eddie, it's not about ignoring the barrier that he's seen; it's about breaking it down, using surfing as a tool.

He explained that he sees the barrier when new participants are hesitant to participate or engage at all, from surfing or even simple conversation. And the reason is often, like Eddie said: these young adults haven't had positive experiences with people who look like him.

But at the end of a surf day, it's completely different.

"The cool thing is that by the end of the day, those are the kids we have to drag out of the water," Eddie said. "I see the barrier breaking down all the time, and nothing makes me happier."

Once that barrier is broken down, mentorship can fill the void where it's needed the most.

I asked Eddie to explain what mentorship looks like, and he was quick to say that it starts with a relationship.

"Mentorship is role modeling and how you act. What you say you're going to do, you do. You mean what you say, and you follow through. That's the heart of MeWater operationally, and it comes from the heart, because Tim and I have mentored kids for decades."

Niki said, "A lot of our kids don't have male figures in their lives or certainly don't have consistent male figures. They don't have a lot of people in their life who say something and deliver. If Eddie promised to take you surfing, he's going to take you surfing and he'll do anything to make it happen."[117]

In addition to relationships, it's not forced. "They will tell us what they want from us, that way we're not being too invasive."

But being a mentor is more than being a surf buddy. "It's not just a day at the beach," Eddie says. "The main point is we are intertwined with the community and families we serve. If someone's grandma calls me and says someone isn't doing what he needs to at home, then I'll get on him. When the kids know you're on the same team as their caregiver, then they understand you're not just 'fun Eddie.' I can take you to the beach, but you need to listen to your grandma."

"He's really made a difference in all of these kid's lives," said Robin Randall, MD, MPH Director of Edgewood Center. "I got to Edgewood 17 years ago. When I got here, Eddie was already here. I've seen kids sort of before and after and that sense of connection to the ocean, that sense of belonging and that sense of sort of calm that comes over them after they master or begin to master surfing is really incredible. Eddie knows how to connect with the kids in ways say, their formal therapist may not be able to or their psychiatrist may not be able to."[118]

The story of MeWater is extraordinary: stepping to fill a void, mentorship, all built around riding a surfboard.

"My dream would be to drive through the neighborhood with this van, and just say come on let's go…Just get the kids to go surfing," Eddie said.

And if you look for Eddie today, that's exactly what you can find him doing.

℮℮℮

From Masi to San Francisco's low income neighborhoods, Chernobyl's surrounding regions and beyond, the challenges that youth populations face daily are complex and dangerous. People like Tim, Apish, Eddie, and Tom have been using surfing to meet those needs, and based on data and testimonials, it's making a difference—one person at a time.

4

TRAUMA THERAPY, VITAMIN SEA & SURF THERAPY FOR WOMEN HEALING FROM TRAUMA

The statistics amongst women experiencing a form of trauma is haunting. Specifically in the United States, 50 percent of women suffer from the negative effects of trauma, 1 in 8 American women will develop clinical depression, 1 in 6 has experienced sexual violence.[119]

What's more, according to the American Psychological Association, women are twice as likely as men to suffer from depression, PTSD, suicidal ideation, and anxiety.[120]

The results of COVID-19 seemed to make these challenges dramatically worse. 83 percent women report a significant increase in depressive symptoms, parental stress, and helplessness due to COVID-19 closures, as compared to 35 percent of men.[121]

The solution, one would imagine, is found in treatment. But, "Half of people in the US who report depression actually seek professional care and traditionally marginalized communities do not access therapy due to a lack of access, histories of oppression, and a lack of trust in the medical system."

Because of this, a few practitioners have pioneered an alternative form of treatment—surf therapy for women healing from trauma. I spoke with organizations helping women escape the horrors of sex trafficking and abuse, as well as refugees. I also spoke with a former pro surfer who, after seeing that women couldn't surf in Muslim nations due to cultural clothing restrictions, decided to pioneer a way of inclusivity for surfing.

Overall, I realized just how big the need is for women healing from trauma—and how surfing is an unlikely source of help.

ℰℰℰ

Natalie Small's surf therapy beginnings were the confluence of several unique factors—the first of which is that the North Carolina native loved to surf.

While working on her MFT marriage and family license in a Masters Program, she felt like something was missing. The entire curriculum focused on talk therapy, though one chapter in a textbook discussed art therapy—something of which Natalie had no idea about. It piqued her interest.

Before completion, Natalie actually stopped her studies and instead began working on boats so that she could travel. She soon earned the title Captain Natalie, and ended up in Argentina where she was hired as a culture shock support person for au pairs. She realized she could get hours towards her license in the process, and looked up a supervisor, who happened to be a proponent of experiential art therapy association for Latin America—Garciela Botoni, the President of the International Expressive Arts Association.

"It turned me back onto what's possible when we welcome our bodies and nature back into the healing process," she told me. Training and mentorship on all forms of art, somatic, and eco therapies followed. Natalie said, "It lit the fire under me that this is possible."

Inspired, she soon returned stateside and started working towards her licenses using art and experiential based therapies and received her licenses.

She was working with Generate Hope, a safehouse for women survivors of sex trafficking, in San Diego. At the house, she led art modalities—ribbon dancing, painting, journaling, creative writing, finger paintings, clay—and one of the questions that kept coming from the participants was what art modality Natalie used for her own mental health.

"The place I always go that has been so consistent my entire life has been the ocean," she said. "I shared with them how surfing had been a big therapist for me and a place I could go for the full range of the human experience, from when I was grieving something, to when I was celebrating something, I was angry, going through a breakup, whatever it was…I could go to the ocean, and she could hold it. I could bring anything to her. Nothing was too big for her to hold and let me work through."

The participants encouraged her to take them to the ocean. After all, she was trained as a surf instructor—and had her lifeguard certifications. "I said I'm sure there's some legal thing around that, I could get my license taken away…But they were persistent, and the house mom gave in and said, 'let's give it a go.'"

In 2012, after pulling together a few surf instructor friends and surfboards from a local surf shop, they scheduled a day at the beach—a day Natalie will never forget.

She explained that in theory, they did art experiential art therapy—but surfing was the paintbrush and the wave was the canvas.

After beach instruction—which included instruction on how to listen to your body and let your body and breath guide you as you learn to surf—the surfing began. Natalie had been working with the women for almost two months, but she noticed a never before seen shift. She gave the example of women who had suffered from sexual trauma and had a disconnection from their bodies: "They were connecting in their body in a whole new way."

"All of a sudden the narrative around their body was transforming from my body was something that has been used, abused and sexualized to my body is strong and feeling alive and empowered. It was completely reframing that in one session."

That wasn't the only change at the beach that Natalie noticed.

"Women were expressing this was the first time they felt joy and laughed since they couldn't even remember. In the house there was a lot of tension between the women, living in the same house dealing with their own recovery, difficulty sharing and connecting…they go into the ocean, and all of a sudden, they're cheering each other on, supporting each other, and getting to be seen."

The therapeutic aspect of the day was enough to show Natalie that surfing was—somehow, some way—working. From that point, Natalie began to run surf therapy sessions—and they began to grow.

"As we were holding those sessions, my girl friends who were surf instructors and volunteers in the water, they saw how amazing it was. They asked if people they knew could come—friends going through postpartum depression, recovering from an eating disorder, in recovery for drug and alcohol abuse, recovering from an abusive relationship, loss of a loved one…The ocean doesn't see what the trauma label is, we're walking the world in, so I thought why not?"

"We had this beautiful intersection of women with different backgrounds and different trauma experiences coming together," Natalie said. "No one knew anyone's trauma story. No one knew we were all there because we've all experienced domestic violence or sexual abuse... we just showed up as a bunch of women to interact and build relationship with our bodies, each other, the ocean, and left those labels on the land. Leaving those labels on the land gave us space to explore the other parts of who we are aside from the traumas we experienced."

While Natalie ran the first surf therapy session in 2012—she describes the first year as "financed by the currency of passion, community, and time"—she didn't have the desire to create an organization. She hoped organizations already existed that she could support by building out a surf therapy curriculum. But with the realization that such didn't exist at the time, coupled with the community's growth, she formally organized it into Groundswell Community Project, a nonprofit, in 2016.

As Natalie ran more and more surf sessions, she was able to further understand the therapy behind it all—and how it mirrored trauma therapy. "It wasn't just a fun sport or activity," she said. "When held with intention, mindfulness and trauma informed therapeutic practices, powerful healing was taking place."

She continued: "From the client's perspective, trauma recovery all of a sudden became joyful. And when something is joyful, you want to keep doing it. It created this sustainable model and it shifted from the client relying on the therapist to the client making community and having community support. In the private practice setting which I was working in, so many clients were dealing with the same stuff and feeling very alone. All of a sudden, being able to come together in community, and recognize 'I'm not alone in this'—not only am I not alone, but I have a whole community of people to surf it with."

She continued: "Rather than it being a processing group, it's a presencing group. In the groups we're not talking trauma stories. That's one of the questions we get beforehand, is 'do I have to tell my trauma story or talk?' You can say nothing for eight weeks of the program and still receive everything. We welcome our bodies to see witness connect and play and the ocean as the co-facilitators to the trauma healing."

But Natalie did realize something that made this alternative form of therapy unique: it was therapeutic for her, as the practitioner as well.

"When we think about trauma healing and therapy, you think this is going to be heavy, I'm going to cry, I'm going to need time afterwards to be ok before I'm around other people. There's this wait and stigma around doing trauma therapy. From being a therapist, I left after doing deep trauma therapy work needing to shake it off and go surfing because I was holding all this stuff from all my clients. After doing a surf therapy session, I was getting my dose of vitamin sea, and getting a chance to be in there and experience the healing benefits of the ocean. As a therapist, from a care provider perspective, it was more sustainable and mentally healthy for me."

Even with Groundswell's growth, Natalie still considered herself a "closest surf therapy provider" because she had a fear that promoting surfing as "therapy" would lead to getting her license taken away.

"In the therapy world, that's a big deal—if 'therapy' doesn't follow regulations, you can get your license taken away. I worked hard to get it, and I didn't want that to happen."

A phone call from Kris Primacio at ISTO calmed Natalie's nerves. "Kris called me and told me that others were doing the same thing—and calling it therapy! She invited me to the conference in South Africa in 2018 and, after that, I realized I can use this term of surf therapy. I owned it, and was thankful for them calling me who I am."

eee

Groundswell's programs include an eight week Surf Sister program, and community drop in programs, which promote ocean safety, surf skills, and tools for trauma recovery, all while being supported by a licensed therapist and trained volunteers.

The goal of both the Surf Sister Program and the drop in programs is that by the end of it, the participants will have three things: tangible tools they learned to improve and maintain a positive mental health, community support, and they know how to access the ocean for their mental health—but not a pro surfer.

"While surfing is the modality of ocean access we utilize, the goal isn't necessarily that everyone walks away a pro surfer. The goal is you find your way of building and connecting with the ocean, your body, and community," Natalie said.

At the end of the day, the goal is a "lifelong wave riding practice for their mental health. Some go on to become strong surfers, others body surf, some swim in the ocean, or even become ocean conservationists or artists expressing their love for the ocean as their medicine and life saver," Natalie said.

The truth is that whatever your age, race or sex, trauma does not discriminate. In order to create equal access and sustainability of the programs, Groundswell provides sliding scale super bills for insurance coverage and full scholarships for participants.

What I found interesting was the former for insurance coverage. "Currently, 'surf therapy' is not recognized by insurance companies as a therapy practice," Natalie said. "But we are working and partnering with private practices, clinics, and research teams to help build the awareness and acknowledgement of surf therapy so in future years insurance forms will include it. For now, we provide super bills and label the surf therapy programs under group therapy for coverage."

It's clear that Groundswell doesn't just facilitate surf therapy; they also facilitate training.

Their introductory Level 1 Training, geared for therapists, students, surf coaches, ocean lovers, examines how surfing can be therapeutic by focusing on "somatic therapeutic modalities."[122]

In their Level 2 Training, of which Level 1 Training is a prerequisite, the training focuses on how to create a safe space for surf therapy, as

well as other mindfulness practices. It's geared for those "actively facilitating or planning to launch surf therapy programs."[123]

They also offer training for surf therapy volunteers, which fills a
large void—volunteering at a surf therapy event can be overwhelming.
This training helps volunteers learn how to be a trauma informed
volunteer in outdoors spaces utilizing nature, their bodies and the
community for healing and support of individuals and communities.

"These classes help legitimize surf therapy practice in the psychology field as well as increase diverse leadership and access to surf therapy,
which is essential to developing a therapy practice that is supportive
and inclusive for all," Natalie said. "That's a big piece of why we started
doing the training and curriculum. All these people were reaching out
and asking how we did it. Surf therapy is the wild west of therapy right
now, and this training helps them learn simple tools, trauma informed
practices, and how organizations can support themselves—and others.
That sustainability is essential."

It's these classes that have had an effect on others around the world
trying to start their own surf therapy program as they've seen the healing
powers of the sea and the need in their local community—including
helping Syrian refugees as they resettle in the United Kingdom.

Today, Natalie continues to lead Groundswell's efforts as surf
therapy—what she called the "wild west"—continues to evolve. She
concluded our conversation by telling me:

> "Indigenous people have been going to the sea for healing since
> humans began…they speak of us all being wave riders as we
> surf our first wave from our mother's womb after spending
> nine months as water beings,' she said. 'Surfing therapy is a
> spiritual practice of coming back home and now, with the
> support of research surf therapy, it can become a recognized
> therapeutic practice that practitioners can be trained in, thus
> creating more safer and braver spaces for individuals and their

communities to reclaim their healing, power, and belonging through reconnecting to the wisdom and medicine of their bodies, community, and the sea. Studies are now starting to prove that the disconnection from these things is the root cause of mental health issues, chronic pain, and disease. Surf therapy brings us back into relationship with all of this and reminds us that healing can actually be joyful. When something is joyful, it is sustainable. When the sea is healthy, we are healthy; when we are healthy our communities are healthy. It is all connected. As I continue to invest my life's work into the development of surf therapy, I'm not just investing in mental health, but also ocean health and community health. They are all interwoven and interdependent."

℮℮℮

Yvette Curtis calls herself an "accidental surf club founder," and it's the confluence of two situations that led to the creation of Wave Wahines, an organization in the United Kingdom that delivers a "trauma informed approach to surfing."[124]

Yvette was working with women in refuge at North Devon Against Domestic Abuse for her own personal reasons and saw a massive need firsthand. At the same time, her daughter wanted to surf, but Yvette couldn't find a club that wasn't competitive, pricey, or had other girls in it; most of them were full of boys.

Because Yvette was looking for a more nurturing environment for her daughter, and because she had seen the need working with women in refuge, she decided to start a surf club—and deliver surf therapy.

She discovered the Groundswell Community Project and, after going through their Level 1 training, was able to get funding for a trial session with her local women's refuge. "It went so well, and the women found it incredible," Yvette told me.

After that, she completed her Level 2 training with Groundswell in order to become a full surf therapy facilitator. Doing so required commitment—because of the time zone, she had to take classes from 2–6 in the morning.

After that, she did two eight-week surf therapy courses with women's refuge, and the testimonials she received were tear jerking, from "you're saving lives" to "you've given me my voice back" and more. At that point, Yvette felt she had found her calling.

Wave Wahines, with the motto "If it doesn't exist—you can make it," was born in 2016.

"Wave Wahines began as a way of getting young women into surfing in an environment that was supportive and inclusive," said Yvette, "and most importantly to show them they don't have to live up to any images of female surfers to get in a wetsuit and on a board. We work so hard to show girls and young women that we are all different and that's what makes us special, that's what makes us powerful, and that's what makes us, us. We are enough. As a community, we should be focusing on empowering the girls of today as they grow into the women of tomorrow by showing them there is another way."

In the years to come, Wave Wahines would exist to help a population who experienced unimaginable trauma.

ℓℓℓ

On the beach in North Devon in the United Kingdom, the tide is high as young girls, ages from 5–11, sit and stand nervously on the beach. Women—moms, grandmothers—dressed in traditional Syrian dresses with their heads covered, watch from afar.

The participants, Syrian refugees who escaped the horrors of civil war and the trauma of being displaced, are here to surf. Some of them had only been in the country for eight weeks.

Because the area of North Devon has a growing population of displaced people resettled through the Community Sponsorship Program—managed by the assistance of the Pickwell Foundation—Yvette saw the needs and also wanted to offer more representative and diverse participation in surfing.

Even though the waves are small—1–2 feet at best—the nerves are high. Not only have none of the girls surfed before; many of them have never been in the ocean before and some don't know how to swim. Beyond that, the girls are still in complete culture shock, and, deep down, are hoping to find acceptance in their new home.

There are no expectations on them: If someone wants to ride in on their board on their belly the whole session, they can. If they want to build sandcastles, they can. If they want to go out of their depth and test their swimming, they can.

They slowly waded out to the sea.

ⓔⓔⓔ

"It was such a moving day," Yvette said, recalling that first surf session with Syrian refugees.

"We initially worked with five girls aged 5–11, and by the end of the final eight weeks, we had nine girls with us following their periods of quarantine—as this first group was at the height of the COVID-19 pandemic in 2020," she said.

What I found interesting was that Yvette thought about who would be delivering the surf therapy beforehand, and how that could impact the population in need. She stipulated that the coaches and volunteers were female "to ensure the families were comfortable with their daughters trying such a new activity with a new group of adults," she said. "I wanted to personally ensure that cultural traditions were respected, and we enabled the girls and their families to feel welcome and accepted."

The language barrier was, well, a barrier. "You don't know what they witnessed, but they can't quite tell you," she said. But surfing—and human kindness—became the universal language.

Yvette told me one of the more powerful moments happened when she tried to communicate through kindness.

She was spending time with a 10-year-old who came to Wave Wahines with her younger sister—their family had only been in the UK eight weeks at that point. To add to the challenges, the family spoke no English, and Yvette only knew a handful of words in Arabic.

"I recall the young girl being incredibly anxious upon arrival and remaining very close to mum in the first instance. As a mum of three myself, I recognized her need for reassurance and offered her my hand and a gentle hello. I was overwhelmed when she took it—a moment of trust from her and responsibility for me. Being older, she would have had a more conscious understanding of the events around her, so her fear of this new experience was one I/we needed to be careful and thoughtful with.

"I held her hand to the shoreline and we didn't enter the water for quite some time. I gestured to her to sit with me on the sand, let the sand fall through our fingers and just experience that feeling.

"After a few minutes, we shuffled closer and repeated that process. We then stood back up and walked until we could let the water touch our feet. The words that kept coming out of my mouth 'I've got you—you're safe' and whilst the words may not have been understandable my tone and holding eye contact and her hands are universal. I will never forget those first few steps into the sea as the small gentle waves bounced against us both and suddenly the fear just fell away and this electric smile lit up her face. Unforgettable and one of the best moments I have ever experienced. Seeing pure joy from real fear was indescribable.

"I am forever grateful for her trust in me at that moment and every second afterward! She returned the following year and is now a proficient swimmer and loves being in the sea! I couldn't be prouder than being able to facilitate that feeling and those moments."

Acting as a translator, one of the mothers on the beach communicated to Yvette and the Wave Wahines volunteers some of the words that the participants described surfing as.

These included:

- Flying
- Happy
- Fun
- Joy
- Free
- Smiling
- Hungry

All words that pointed to one notion: surf therapy was helping.

In 2022, Yvette was able to grow the program, which included providing transport to the sea, along with a surf session for boys.

"We will be continuing to drive this program forwards and show how surfing and the water can be a real tool for healing, resilience and community for displaced peoples," Yvette told me.

Yvette is also removing the clothing barrier that prevents many Syrian refugees from surfing. Because Muslim women are traditionally required to cover their head, neck, and the majority of their body, getting in the water to surf can be a barrier in itself.

That's why Yvette is utilizing a new clothing option—born from a female pro surfer traveling to Iran and seeing the need firsthand—so the women don't have any barriers to climb, only waves to surf.

An Ireland native, Easkey Britton has a historic relationship with the sea. Her grandmother, Mary Britton, a hotel owner, returned to Ireland from a trip to California determined to bring two Malibu surfboards back to her local beach—Rossnowlagh. Since she was a hotel owner, she had planned on offering them to guests, but instead, her five sons— Easkey's father Barry included—took the boards to the waves, making the Britton boys some of the first pioneers of Irish surfing.[125]

Thus, Easkey was born into a surfing family and took the passion to be her own. She competed as part of the Irish surf team, representing Ireland at the European Junior and Senior Championships and World Surfing Games for many years and is the first Irish person to be nominated for the Global WSL Big Wave Awards. After pro surfing, she began free surfing—traveling around the globe in search of waves and adventure and documenting it all.

In 2010, she, along with French filmmaker Marion Poizeau ventured to Baluchestan in Southern Iran in search of empty and uncharted surf. Located between Pakistan and the gulf of Oman, the area saw swell for a few months a year during the Indian monsoon season. But after that, it would disappear like a mirage.

In Iran, as a consequence of the Islamic Revolution in 1979, many aspects of women's lives became dictated by the state, including compliance with compulsory hijab (head covering) laws when in public spaces.

To physically get into the ocean, Easkey had to be covered from head to toe, in order to comply with the legal requirement for all women to be hijab-compliant. A wetsuit would be too hot under the intense desert sun as well as too figure-hugging, and in the absence of any modest full-body surf-wear for women, she wore baggy boardshorts over sports leggings, a long sleeved rashvest, a loose fitting shirt over everything and a scarf for a makeshift hijab. Not only was this uncomfortable; it was restrictive and potentially dangerous. Once saturated with saltwater, the hijab would get heavy and could make it hard to breathe, especially after duck diving—or wiping out. In addition to this, all of this clothing in a region that regularly experiences temperatures well over 30 degrees Celsius—86 degrees Fahrenheit—during the summer season, resulted in significant sweating, which could lead to the dangerous effects of dehydration.

Marion captured Easkey surfing fun-sized, clean, and empty desert waves while surfing fully covered and receiving an overwhelming positive response from crowds of local people who gathered on the beach to watch the spectacle of surfing for the first time. And the first surfer they saw was a woman. "I didn't realize at the time the impact that would have," Easkey said.

Three years later, after connecting online with pioneering Iranian female athletes, snowboarder Mona Seraji and swimmer and diver Shahla Yasini, Easkey returned to the area along with Mona and Shahla to introduce them to surfing for the first time. The historic moment when the young Iranian women, along with local Baluch youth Shams Fuladi, became the pioneers of surfing in their country was captured by Marion in the award-winning documentary *Into the Sea*. "That was the turning point in my relationship with the ocean and understanding what surfing could be as a vehicle for connection and change," Easkey said.

Over the coming years, in collaboration with Iran's first female triathlete Shirin Gerami and local women, Easkey returned to the coast of Baluchestan each summer to deliver training workshops and co-facilitate a programme called Be Like Water—an active, physical practice aimed at tapping into the more playful, creative and therapeutic qualities of water and the sea. It was a way to help make surfing more accessible for minority groups of women and girls in Iran, especially those who had never had access to the water before, and, according to Easkey, "to support a greater body-self-nature connection." The performance aspect of learning to surf—paddle, paddle paddle!—was replaced with a focus on embodiment practices—that active process of self-discovery (e.g. connecting with breath, moving like water, body surfing), and in effect, teaching participants "water dancing rather than surfing."[126]

Easkey wrote of the experience:

> *"This was not about challenging traditional customs that could lead to polarization or opposition from others before we even got started. Instead, it was about celebration, celebrating the beauty in our differences, so that the way women and girls saw themselves changed. Changing their self-image is a crucial transforming force for women and girls."[127]*

Easkey collected all her thoughts, experiences and recommendations in *'Be Like Water': Reflections on Strategies Developing Cross-Cultural Programmes for Women, Surfing and Social Good*, which was published in the The Palgrave Handbook of Feminism and Sport, Leisure and Physical Education in 2018.

Following these experiences – witnessing and actively participating in the beginning of the development of surfing in Iran for both male and female surfers, Easkey knew clothing would remain a limiting factor for female surfers unless she could help find a solution. She connected with Finisterre, a British surf brand that designs functional and sustainable product for those that share a love of the sea.[128]

"Easkey came home telling us what an amazing experience she had in Iran and that there was a growing interest to do this activity, but that there was a barrier," explains Finisterre's Product Director, Debbie Luffman. "It was the perfect design problem. Not only was it a functional problem, but the clothing was actually stopping you from doing or enjoying the activity you wanted to do."[129]

The result of their collaboration is a full-coverage seasuit and surf hijab designed to enable access for all, empowering a diversity of women with the choice of what they want to wear.

- The Into the Sea Seasuit is a full-coverage swimsuit that provides full body coverage without being skin-tight, can easily be worn over a wetsuit if needed, and provides SPF 50+ protection.[130]
- The Into The Sea Hijab is a securely fitting swim Hijab. The head covering is strategically designed to provide coverage and stay put in rough seas, whether swimming or surfing and is also ideal for general exercise. It too offers SPF 50+ protection.[131]

Debbie echoed Easkey's sentiment that the goal of the suit was to help women experience surfing, not make a political statement. "We wanted to be really mindful not to trample on anyone's culture—who are we to impose ourselves on that? We were much more interested in the functional barrier."[132]

Thanks to these efforts, and the growth of surfing as a whole, Iran has a growing surf scene where men can surf, but also women—offering a powerful sense of embodiment, self-connection and self-actualization, as well as connection to the power of the Ocean, all of which have been shown to aid recovery and healing from trauma.

Easkey voiced this impact by saying: "One woman recently wrote to me from Iran: 'I finally understood the most important skill to surf, connection with Mother Ocean. Believe it or not it changed my whole being.'"[133]

But that's not all. One of the many young women Easkey helped to surf, Farima Nouri, became the first female in Iran to be awarded a surf scholarship by the International Surfing Association (ISA) in 2018.

"With the support and encouragement of some of Iran's early female pioneers of surfing who help local youth apply for the ISA scholarship every year, a local girl has been a recipient of the almost award every year since helping to boost the visibility and social acceptance locally and nationally of the importance of surfing for women and girls," Easkey said. The following year, Venous Balouch became the youngest female recipient aged 8, laying the foundations for the continued growth of female surfing in the country.

In recent years, Easkey has surfed with women wearing the Finisterre creations at the Wave—the wavepool located inland in Bristol, England—showing not only can it allow you to surf, but you can wear it and absolutely rip.

Easky said: "For those who have overcome the barriers, the sense of freedom through something like surfing in the sea can be powerful and linked to our fundamental need for recognition, equality, and identity. It can allow us to expand after years of being conditioned to contract."[134]

Today, Easkey, who has a PhD, and is the author of several books, including Saltwater in the Blood and Ebb & Flow, continues to advocate for surf therapy—and a connection with the ocean.

"We are a traumatized society, one could argue," she told me. "There's so much trauma and layers of it. We have crippled health care systems here in the West, under a lot of pressure. Surf therapy is still considered fringe but I'm seeing it shift globally and here in Ireland. As a blue health researcher, I support local surf therapy charity, Liquid Therapy to evidence the impact of their programmes so they can better communicate the benefits of connecting with the ocean for our well-being, especially mental health. The more traditional health services have started to include surf therapy in their social prescribing for the first time since 2022. This could help create a cultural shift in how we relate to and connect with nature, restoring planetary health, a sense of stewardship, and enhancing ocean literacy."

ᥫᥫᥫ

While living in Hawaii and serving as the Editor of Freesurf Magazine, I interviewed a well-known waterman named Brian Keaulana—I would argue a living legend—on the sands of Makaha Beach on Oahu's west side. As clean, head high surf filled into the arena, Brian was talking about ocean safety, and working with not just Hawaii but also other countries to help them boost their ocean safety efforts as well.

"We're not divided by land, but connected by water," he told me.

That quote has stuck with me ever since—and it rings so true with Natalie, Yvette and Easkey.

"I went through my whole journey and process and struggles and failures and to start Groundswell," Natalie told me. "If others can utilize that to stand on my shoulders and go further versus them figure it out on their own—that's my hope."

Natalie's training from Groundswell have reverberated across the Atlantic Ocean to Yvette and became the catalyst for healing amongst female Syrian refugees. And it's Easkey's efforts, combined with Finisterre, that led to more inclusivity among women in Iran, at The Wave in England, and around the world.

To add onto Brian's original quote, the surf therapy community isn't divided by land—it's obvious they are connected by water.

5

INCARCERATION, DRUG ADDICTION & HOW TO "LIVE FOR MORE"

A t 10am on a cool Tuesday morning, a group of surf instructors and male participants, all wearing brightly colored turquoise and white rashguards that say, "Live For More," form a circle in the sand on Omanu Beach in Mount Maunganui, a beautiful stretch of white sand found on the North Island of New Zealand.

All eyes and ears inside the colorful circle are on Krista Davis. Everything about her is bright: her blonde hair, her green eyes, her white smile. The goal for her today—and the organization she founded called Live for More, which officially launched in 2016—is simple: use surfing as a way to engage with young men, ages 17-25, caught up in the lifestyles of drugs, alcohol, gangs, prison, violence, or anything else that society labels "negative" or "too hard to deal with."

She asks how everyone is both mentally and physically on a scale of 1–10. After everyone provides an answer, she explains how this surf session is going to work: every male participant will be paired up with a surf instructor. For those who are beginners, the instructor will help line them up with the waves and give them a push. For the participants who are more experienced, the instructors will surf alongside them, giving them tips to improve their new skill.

Krista pauses to glance at the wave conditions, and for a moment, the only noise on the empty beach is the crashing of stomach high swells in the distance. The glassy waves break underneath the rising sun, shining light so bright that it's causing the young men in the circle to squint.

After the beach instruction ends, the instructors and participants each pick up a foam surfboard off the sand and walk towards the waterline. One of those instructors is Jared Dixon.

Even though he can seem intimidating at first glance—he has broad, strong shoulders, deep brown eyes, and a steady and confident gait—his tone is friendly as he talks with the participant he's assigned to surf with. The tide washes over their feet as they watch as an incoming set build, and Jared offers a few quick tips to the young man. As the tide pulls back, the wet sand reflects their smiling faces backlit by the golden morning light.

They jump in, their wetsuits providing warmth from the cool ocean temperature, and begin paddling towards the area the waves are breaking along with the rest of the group. Once they reach the lineup, they sit on their boards, and like everyone else, focus on the bright horizon.

A building set approaches, Jared tells the participant to get ready, and as the wave nears, he yells to begin paddling—*hard*. When Jared sees the participant slowly rise above the crashing whitewash and glide on the wave towards shore, he lets out a cheer that reverberates throughout the lineup, the same cheer that Krista and other surf instructors are making watching other participants.

This scene plays on repeat for the next hour. The highlight of the morning is the entire group, both surf instructors and participants, catching a party wave, gliding towards shore together. For anyone watching the party wave from the beach on this Tuesday morning, it looks like a surf camp. But it's far more than that.

Most of the surfers on the party wave are Māori, the native people of New Zealand. Māori are overrepresented in nearly every negative statistic in New Zealand. According to Krista, the Māori make up just 15 percent of the country's population, yet they make up roughly 51 percent of the prison population. The majority of Live For More's participants have already been a part of that 51 percent, previously imprisoned for committing violent crimes, such as assault, and/or using and selling drugs, like methamphetamine.

"There's not a lot of support for this demographic," Krista tells me. "A lot of people dump them in the 'too hard' basket. The sad thing is that most of them are desperate to change, they just don't know how. They've had no positive role models. There's talk of these young people who fall through the cracks; these young people are born in the cracks. Its generational cycles of neglect, abuse, drug use, gang involvement, in and out of prison, poverty, and lack of education."

When I learned that the organization uses surfing to change these generational cycles of drug abuse and imprisonment, I was curious how the simple act of riding a wave could be so powerful.

After the hour-long surf session at Omanu Beach, the group carries the surfboards back up to the parking lot. They each change clothes, and the participants have a smoke break. But this smoke break is different from the first one, which took place before they formed a colorful circle on the beach. The air during the first smoke break was quiet and reserved, the young men keeping to themselves. Now, the group is full of energy and excitement, sharing their stories from taming waves in the wild sea. Jared listens and smiles as he helps other instructors neatly stack the foam surfboards in a trailer.

Once the surfboards are loaded, the group gets back into vehicles and heads towards the second half of the day—lunch followed by several group therapy discussions.

During one of those discussions, they again form a circle, but this time on couches with a surfboard-shaped coffee table in the middle. Today, it's Jared's turn to speak. What he begins to say sounds shockingly similar to what each of the young men are going through at the moment. He knows the pull of addiction. He knows the loneliness of prison. He explains to the young men in the circle that had he never paddled out on a Live for More surfboard alongside Krista, he wouldn't be sitting here on the couches sharing his story. He might still be in prison.

Or worse, he might not even be alive.

ℓℓℓ

Aggravated robbery landed Jared in a New Zealand prison for the first time. Laying under a bright white light in his cell, surrounded by four white walls, the 18-year-old wondered how he got to this point.

Stealing began at a young age for Jared—lollipops, chocolates, even eggs to throw at cars. "We were poor," he told me. "I think coming from not a rich family, not having a lot, we saw people had stuff that we sort of needed or wanted, and there was only one way to get it—we had to steal it for ourselves."

Along with stealing, he was also introduced to addiction at a young and formative age. In "The Drop: How the Most Addictive Sport Can Help us Understand Addiction and Recovery," Thad Ziolkowski writes "addiction sprouts and grows over time in the sunlight and soil of certain conditions—genetic, personal, cultural."[135] Jared grew up in soil ripe for addiction. He had no positive role models in his life. What's more, his family encouraged drug use, like marijuana. At the age of 16, he used meth for the first time.

Along with stealing and addiction came gang ties, which he inherited from his family. It was in a gang where Jared found his community, where he found his tribe.

Out of these three dangerous and deadly activities, the first that had him in trouble with the law was stealing. Stealing lollipops and chocolates evolved into stealing cars and robbing and assaulting people. Arrested and charged with aggravated robbery, he was sentenced to two and a half years in the New Zealand prison system. Jared spent that time surrounded by four white walls in his cell, and when the door opened, he congregated with those who had similar offenses, gang ties and drug addictions.

Before the end of his prison sentence, Jared was paroled, and as part of the agreement, he was to meet with a counselor. He was introduced to Krista, and in between four walls, they talked about the challenges he faced.

At the time, Krista was fulfilling her passion of helping people with addiction by working as a counselor. But she saw limitations with traditional therapy trapped inside four walls. Some would miss sessions, and for those who came, it took multiple sessions across multiple weeks to build rapport. A surfer, Krista wondered if wave riding could help these boys. After taking a few participants surfing, she discovered that it became a vehicle to engage with what she calls "hard to engage guys."

After talking with Krista, Jared, now in his early 20s, decided to sign up for the surf program. But just a week before his first surf session, he wanted something that he didn't have. There was only one way, his ingrained habits told him, to get it: rob someone. He was again charged with aggravated robbery. But this time, there would be no option for parole. He had to serve a sentence of over three years in its entirety.

Jared was back staring at four walls, wondering how he got there. One day, he received a letter. "To everyone in jail, getting letters is like a birthday present," he told me. It was from Krista offering words of encouragement and support. Over the next three years, the letters kept coming, keeping him "hopeful" for a future better than his past. After completing his prison sentence and walking out of jail, one of the first things on his list was surfing.

What was once Krista taking participants surfing was now Live For More, a charitable trust, with three programs. The first, called Tai Ora, translates to "waves of change," and serves as an introduction for the participant to the organization and vice versa. Next is Tai Wātea ("waves of freedom"), an intensive 9 to 10 week program that includes surf therapy, clinical counseling, life navigation, youth mentoring and more. Third is Tai Tautoko ("waves of support"), an ongoing form of support, helping participants who have graduated Tai Wātea stay on track, a relapse prevention type of support.

Jared committed to everything that Live For More had to offer, and after sitting in the circle at a beach known as Shark Alley for beach instruction, Krista acted as his surf instructor and pushed him into his first wave. When remembering the day, Jared told me that he didn't want help surfing. "I wanted to do it myself," he said with a laugh. "I had waited for this day for years to take him surfing," Krista said while showing me a photo from the day: Jared with a surfboard in hand along with other participants. Jared looked at the photo and admitted that he was still on drugs at the time. But he also said that during that surf session, he felt powerful emotions that he hadn't felt before. A rush of adrenaline. Happiness. Joy. Peace. Jared was instantly hooked on surfing, and those closest to him saw an instant difference.

"When the program started and he had his first surf, if I ever needed evidence of how this program impacts young men, he was my proof," Kerry-Anne Winders, his probation officer, said in the documentary film *Waves of Freedom*. "I just remember going out to meet him at the office, it was the afternoon after his first surf. The way he was standing, he was taller... shoulders back, head up, chin up, beaming with this big smile like he was sparkling. He was just a different person all together after one day out in the surf."[136]

Krista agreed that there was something immediately different about Jared after just one surf session. "That first day that we took him surfing, he was a different young guy after that," she said. "Even his probation officer who he caught up with the afternoon of his first day surfing, she sent me this email that was like 'what have you done with him? He came in here today a totally different young man. His head was higher. He stood taller. He looked me in the eyes. He was happy. He was joyful.' She and his psychologist had both been really worried about him, because even in his first month since he had been released, he was just going down. And they were like 'what are we going to do...' They were feeling a bit helpless as to how to support him. And they saw this massive transformation in him in one day of surfing."[137]

Within the programs is a points system, where participants can earn a hat, hoodie, and even a surfboard for certain behaviors and achievements. Jared wanted his own surfboard, but his old habits of stealing wouldn't work in this setting. Instead, he had to earn it. Achievement by achievement, he did just that: Live For More presented him with a bright green surfboard that was his to keep. He had no idea that it was this bright green surfboard that would help save his life in the months to come.

eee

Jared took the lessons he had learned—lessons to help him "live for more"—home after he graduated Tai Wātea. While these new lessons were imprinted on his mind, they still needed time to set, like the ink of a permanent tattoo. In the meantime, the habits that were tattooed many years prior in his mind soon surfaced.

His use of alcohol, marijuana and meth returned, growing heavier than ever before. His involvement with the gangs became more frequent than ever before. Returning back to his old ways while aware of new ways he learned through Live For More put him in a spiraling depression. "I felt like my soul had been taken away from the drugs, gang tension, my upbringing," he said.[138]

Soon, it all came to a head. After coming down from a meth high, Jared found himself in a depressive state. He looked at his surroundings and realized he wasn't just sitting on a couch in his parents' garage, a place where he slept; He was at rock bottom. At that moment, Jared believed that his life was going to go in one of two directions: he was going to go back to jail, or because of gang violence, he was going to be killed. Then, he saw something, something that offered a third option he hadn't previously thought of—the bright green Live for More surfboard he had earned.

"I saw my bright green surfboard. I looked at it and I sort of felt... positive," Jared said. "I felt alive again. I knew this surfboard was going to bring me happiness; I wanted that feeling back. That freedom. That peace. I knew that surfboard was going to bring me peace and freedom. I was just hugging it."

Live For More came to his mind, and even though he had graduated out of the program, he decided to send the organization a text asking for help. After pressing send, Jared, in tears, his arms wrapped around his surfboard, waited.

ℓℓℓ

To understand what Jared was facing at this critical moment in his life, staring at a decision between life and death while hugging a bright green surfboard, I wanted to better understand the generational lifestyle he was trapped in.

I learned that while New Zealand is known for its breathtaking national parks and pristine beaches, the nation also has a darker side—it's known for a shocking amount of meth use, high gang rates, and one of the highest imprisonment rates in the developed world.[139]

Let's start with what Jared was addicted to at this point in his life—meth. At a per capita level, New Zealand has one of the highest rates of meth consumption in the world.[140] A recent study found that "over half of all prisoners (56 percent) had used methamphetamine at some time during their lives and, of those who had used it, over half (58 percent) had used it in the previous 12 months."[141]

"The problem is as bad, if not worse, than ever," said Jared Savage, a senior journalist for the New Zealand Herald and author of *Gangland: New Zealand's Underworld of Organised Crime*. "Meth gives an incredible high, especially the first time it is consumed; the drug stimulates a user's central nervous system to release huge amounts of dopamine, which in turn makes people feel energetic, attractive, intelligent, alert, and talkative. Meth also increases sex drive. So, I can see why it is attractive for people who might be experimenting, but also as an escape for those whom I might describe as living in deprivation."

Because of Jared's upbringing, it's easy to see him fitting into the portrait that Jared Savage paints, a scene of someone in deprivation seeking an escape.

The popularity of gangs—and that Jared inherited ties to them—made his situation even more challenging. Due to colonization, the Māori in New Zealand are without their native land, their native community, and their native identity. What fills the void are modern day tribes, otherwise known as gangs. New Zealand has one of the highest gang membership rates in the world, so high that cumulatively, gang groups are larger than the country's army.[142] But it's not just the quantity that makes gangs dangerous; it's the gang warfare that Jared was so concerned about.

Meth used as an escape, ties to dangerous gangs…On top of these, not only does New Zealand have one of the highest imprisonment rates in the developed world;[143] Māori, like Jared, are overrepresented at every stage in the criminal justice system.

One study found that Māori are 37 percent of people prosecuted by police; 45 percent of people convicted are Māori, and 52 percent of people in prison are Māori. This is despite Māori being only approximately 15 percent of the New Zealand population.[144]

To help understand just how dramatic this is, consider this: a separate study found that Māori currently make up 51.7 percent of the prison population, which equates to a 3.5 times over-representation per capita. The racial disparities are less for African Americans in the United States, who are over-represented in the US prison population by 2.8 times.[145]

Take a deeper look into the high percentage of imprisoned Māori and you'll discover many of them are, like Jared, young: around 34 percent of the prison population are between the ages of 20 and 29.[146]

Even worse, reoffending rates are high, pointing to a systemic issue. Around 70 percent of people with previous convictions are reconvicted within two years following their release from prison. Around 49 percent are re-imprisoned after two years following release from prison.[147]

All of these statistics, studies and reports gave a forewarning as to what was going to happen next for Jared as he waited on a couch in a garage, his arms wrapped around his bright green surfboard and tears running down his face.

But what the statistics didn't factor in was the therapeutic power of surfing.

ぐぐぐ

Krista's phone buzzed. She opened it and saw the message Jared had sent—it was an SOS. She immediately dropped what she was doing, asked a Live for More coworker for help, and the two headed in the direction of Jared's house as quickly as they could.

"Jared had been on our radar for ages because we knew he was really, really, really, *really* struggling," Krista said. "We kept reaching out to him heaps. Sometimes he would engage, sometimes he wouldn't. We kept saying 'we're here when you're ready.' I had no idea what situation we were going to arrive to at his house."

When they arrived, they told one of his family members that Jared had messaged them asking for help. His family didn't know where he was, but they eventually found him in the shed—"the garage, as you guys would say [in America]," Krista said—and what Krista saw broke her heart.

"He was sitting on his couch next to his surfboard so broken. So broken. Just crying; I've never seen Jared cry before. So defeated. We just sat there with him. I don't think much was said. Someone in his family walked in and said, 'Let's go have a session, you just need to get high' and my coworker and I realized we needed to get him away from there. We brought him back to the office and made a plan for what we were going to do. It was the turning point. All of a sudden, Jared said 'I want to change. I'm sick of this.' If he hadn't messaged us and we hadn't gone, then it could be a very different story. We could have lost Jared. We've lost one of our boys to suicide before."

Jared's decision to make a change—and reaching out to Live for More for help to accomplish that—spoke volumes to both Krista and his probation officer, Kerry-Anne. It was like getting back on the surf-board after a head-first wipeout.

"For people like Jared, with addiction issues and things like that, there's always periods of lapses," Kerry-Anne said.[148] "You have to expect that they're going to fall over at some point and if they can pick themselves back up and get back on track, that's what we're after. That's the bit we need to see. That they know what they're doing because a lapse is actually normal. We always just hope that lapse doesn't become so huge that it becomes a relapse so they carry on that way for a period of time too long. Or that the lapse is going to involve some serious offending, obviously."

Jared swam up from the sandy bottom of the ocean, jumped back on the surfboard, and paddled back out for another wave, figuratively and literally. He met with a pastor, who asked him if he wanted to give up drugs, gangs, and give his life to Christ. He said yes and became a Christian. "God freed me from drugs, alcohol, cigarettes," he said. Ever since that day, Jared has been clean.

Today, Jared is a youth mentor with Live For More. He acts as a surf instructor and fills a crack with the organization, a crack that he himself fell into. "Jared's role is huge," Krista said. "Participants graduate, and a lot of them still need heaps of support. We realized we needed someone to keep working with these guys because they come from 25 years of dysfunction and that doesn't change in 10 weeks. With Jared starting with us as a full-time mentor, the guys get a lot of more support now. Jared backslid. If someone does as well as Jared does and then backslides, Jared understands it because he's done that. Jared's big role is supporting the graduates in a lot of ways."

Krista tells me that just as they were always there for Jared, the organization is always there for their participants, even those who have graduated Tai Watea; all are welcome to sit in a circle on Omanu Beach and paddle out alongside Jared through the Tai Tautoko program.

During our conversation, Krista pointed out just how impactful Jared is to the organization, a living and breathing testimony of their program. While many young men in the program hear Jared's story for the first time when he shares it sitting on couches, a few sometimes recognize him from his past life—they bought, used, and sold drugs with Jared.

"It's been quite powerful because they know where he used to be and how bad it used to be, and then they see him now and they're like 'what the heck'…it gives them a lot of hope," Krista said. "Jared has the ability to reach these guys in a way that no one here at Live for More can reach them."

Jared's words and actions collectively have one simple yet powerful message at Live For More: if I can do this, so can you.

eee

I first heard Jared's story at the 2019 International Surf Therapy Organization (ISTO) Conference. The reality that surfing could help young men escape the deadly rip current of drugs, alcohol, gangs, and prison was shocking—and equally inspiring. The image of Jared hugging his surfboard while in the depths of depression and drug addiction has stuck with me ever since.

Although Jared told me that surfing brought him feelings of freedom and peace, I asked him to elaborate more on how standing on a piece of foam in the ocean has been therapeutic throughout his beautiful journey.

"It's a cleansing when I get in the water," he said. "Whatever is on my mind…how I'm feeling…I would let the water take it all away. It's a sort of cleansing. Just a wash over me. It just cleans my mind out."

What Jared may not have realized is that there's more than just feeling a sort of cleansing when surfing. There's something that happens in his brain when he surfs that, in part, answers how surfing has been therapeutic for him—and for others facing what he conquered.

Let's rewind to that first time Jared surfed, soon after being released from his second stint for aggravated robbery in prison. As he jumped into the cool aqua water, paddled out on his first surf session and Krista pushed him into his first wave, something unique happened in his brain.

In what's called the limbic system, the act of standing up on a board causes dopamine—a feel good neurotransmitter that helps our brain understand reward-type behavior that's necessary for survival, such as eating—to be released. Inside the limbic system, you can find neurons, which exist to transmit electrical impulses and chemical signals between different areas of the brain. Dopamine traveled from one of his neurons across a small gap—what's called a synapse—into a neighboring neuron. As Jared glided towards shore on wave, this release gave him an instant good feeling, a euphoria, also known as "runner's high." As he fought to keep his balance on the board, the dopamine transporters quickly removed the dopamine from the neuron, which is the brain's way of preventing the neurons from becoming overstimulated from too heavy of a dose.

After many waves and many dopamine hits, Jared exited the water and felt what he described as "freedom" and "peace." What he didn't realize was that biologically, he was feeling a highly addictive dopamine rush. He was hooked on surfing.

In "Blue Mind: The Surprising Science That Shows How Being Near, In, On, or Under Water Can Make You Happier, Healthier, More Connected, and Better at What You Do," scientist Wallace J Nichols writes about this addictive surfing experience:

> "...Dopamine release is associated with novelty, risk, desire, and effort activity; it's also a key part of the system by which the brain learns. All of these factors, Zald points out, are present in surfing: 'as surfers are first learning, there's an amazing burst of dopamine simply when they stand on the board...Novelty? Check. Risk? Check. Learning? Check. Aerobic activity? Check. Dopamine? In spades." But that's not all...aerobic exercises (such as surfing) produce endorphins, the opioids that affect the prefrontal and limbic areas of the brain involved in emotional processing, and create the feeling of euphoria, known as runner's high. The beauty of the natural environment where people surf also increases the sense of a peak emotional experience. Add the dopamine, the endorphins, and the natural setting to the adrenaline rush produced by the amygdala's fight or flight impulse

when a surfer is faced with a large wave (or a wave of any kind when you're first starting out), and you've got a seriously addictive experience."[149]

Now, let's compare Jared's brain on surfing to Jared's brain on meth by fast forwarding to his relapse after graduating the Tai Wātea program. When meth entered his system, similar to surfing, it caused a dopamine release from neurons across the synapse and into neighboring neurons. But what makes meth so dangerous—and so addicting—is that it strategically blocks the dopamine transporters from doing their jobs to remove the dopamine.

Thus, more and more dopamine is released, and with nowhere for the extreme amount of dopamine to go, Jared's synaptic cells went into overdrive, giving him an intense and euphoric meth high. But this wasn't sustainable. With all of his feel-good neurotransmitters depleted, he fell into a depressive state, and found himself at rock bottom. Then, he looked at his bright green surfboard. At that moment, he remembered feelings of happiness, peace, and freedom—the feel-good dopamine release—and realized that surfing could be his way out. That, in combination with Live For More's willingness to help him, saved his life.

On his road to recovery, Jared had access to something that many recovering addicts don't: the ability to still get that thrill, that dopamine rush that drugs provide. In place of drugs was a far more healthy, natural, and sustainable option—surfing.

But this begs the question: can surfing provide the same high as meth? I asked Dr. Howard Fields, the founder of the University of California at San Francisco Pain Management Center. Dr. Fields' group was the first to demonstrate the clinical effectiveness of opioids for neuropathic pain, and today, his work continues to focus on the "neurobiology of opioid reward."[150]

Dr. Fields explained to me that because we haven't put expensive brain scanners on surfers before they paddle out, and because we don't have the ability to study a surfer's brain on a wave through imaging like a MRI, we don't know the answer to this question—yet. So, I asked him a more general question: can surfing *really* be a replacement for recovering drug abusers?

"I think that's an easy question and the answer is yes, I do," he said. "There's very good evidence, for example, that for some people who are addicted, you can actually get them to take less drugs by paying them to take less drugs. It's what they call contingency therapy. You give someone something that moves their decision making away from the drug and towards something that's not as self-destructive."

He explained that most of today's treatment for drug abuse falls under the auspices of "harm reduction," which prevents the physical harm that the drug can cause. For example, Narcan blocks or reverses the effects of opioids; giving it to someone who overdoses can save their life. "People in the addiction medicine field think these are real treatments," he said. While Narcan can save a life, it won't address the root cause of the addiction that may cause the next overdose.

"The only thing that is going to ultimately work is giving somebody something they prefer to do rather than take the drug," Dr. Fields told me. "In my mind, there's no question a significant proportion of people with drug addiction can be helped by the kind of behavioral approaches that would include things like surfing."

ᥱᥱᥱ

Yes, Jared was hooked on surfing, but I learned there was more to Live For More than just riding a wave. Within its programs are additional exercises that worked to address the root cause of his addiction.

These exercises helped Jared reimagine his identity. Krista designed the Live for More program to emphasize Māori participant's true tribe—not their gang tribe. "So many of our boys come to us and they lack identity and a strong foundation of who they are, which is why they went to the gangs," she said. "We're empowering them and getting them confident. They're not just a druggie, they're not just a gang member, they're not just a thug…they are young men who have a history, culture and identity in New Zealand."

She continued: "People in jail often have little connection to culture to their native tongue, so there's a huge disconnect. We're trying to bridge that to build their confidence, sense of self and pride, also build their identity and who they are. So many of them are lost and floating, and other identities are grabbing them that aren't actually their true ones."

Live For More addresses this disconnect by teaching participants a haka, a ceremonial dance that is intended to display a tribe's pride and strength, along with their "pepeha," a family tree that explains how the person is related to their Māori ancestors. A pepeha is spoken when you introduce yourself. For example, when Jared introduces himself, he says:

Ko Mauao te maunga (Mount Maunganui is my mountain)

Ko Tauranga te moana (Tauranga is my ocean)

Ko Takitimu te waka (Takitimu is my boat)

Ko Ngāti Ranginui te iwi (Ngāti Ranginui is my tribe)

Ko Ngai te Ahi te hapu (Ngai te Ahi is my sub-tribe)

Ko Hairini te marae (Hairini is my meeting place)

Ko Jared Dixon toku ingoa (My name is Jared Dixon)

When I asked how impactful learning his pepeha was, Jared said, "learning about who I am and where I'm from lifted me and gave me stability and foundation that helped me get to where I am now."

After learning about the addictive cocktail of surfing, how it can be a replacement therapy for drug abusers and how cultural exercises can help participants reimagine their identity, I began to see why Live For More can help participants that society labels "negative" or "too hard to deal with" experience true life change.

But what became most profound of all was they had data to back it all up.

eee

"Oh, you're just taking people surfing."

This is the reaction Krista has received when she shares about Live For More's programs. It's the same stigma that other surf therapists around the world voiced to me as well. But the organization has the proof behind the power of their therapy—both measurable and unmeasurable.

In the category of measurable, Annericke Pretorius, a surf therapy researcher, conducted a study among Live For More participants. In the first ever surf therapy study in New Zealand,[151] she found fascinating results. She told me:

> "This study was the first to examine the effects of a surf therapy program on primarily justice-involved young men and the first study to investigate surf therapy outcomes within New Zealand. The year-long study showed that 25 out of 27 participants demonstrated statistically significant improvement in their psychological and social functioning, with 20/27 showing clinically significant improvement as well (this means going from functioning at a clinically unwell level to a level of normal functioning as an 'everyday man on the street'). "In addition, the study showed that many participants reported a reduction in suicidal ideation and drug and alcohol use after attending the program. This is significant, as Māori males between 15-25 are at highest risk of suicide, a risk increased again by AOD consumption. Lastly, the study also showed that the Tai Wātea program has a lower non-completion percentage (20 percent) than other community-based programs

for offenders (40 percent). These findings indicate that the Tai Wātea surf therapy program is a highly promising and valuable therapeutic avenue for improving the psychosocial functioning of hard-to-reach, high-risk young males residing in New Zealand."

What struck me was a 74 percent success rate[152] for participants making the transformation from "clinically unwell" to functioning "as an everyday man on the street"—a success rate that traditional therapies for this population rarely see.

And that's another aspect that I asked Krista about—how participants respond to Live For More's programs compared to traditional therapy. Given that she had previously worked in traditional therapy, she could easily see the differences.

"The guys showed up about 50 percent of the time and it took many sessions to develop a strong rapport. You saw them for one hour each week," she said, discussing traditional therapy. "But with this program, we see them eight hours on one day, plus one hour sessions on separate days, so the rapport you build—especially outside of the office, just doing life with them, activities, sport, laughing, running around, playing touch rugby, surfing, etc.—is amazing, and quick. Surf therapy can provide much more bang for buck and the return is heaps more than 'traditional' support."

She continued: "The guys we are working with honestly would not show up for other things or get the support they desperately need. But at Live for More, they feel safe, they trust, they feel comfortable, there is a brotherhood, and this then allows for vulnerability and healing and so much more."

Even with the data, there are immeasurables with surf therapy. Krista explained that one participant breaking the generational cycle can help older family members do the same; it can also help the young man's children, for example, not inherit gang ties.

"You can't really measure the actual impact," she said. "We've had family members come to us and say 'you've saved my son's life, and because of this, his brother is doing better, you've restored our relationship and now I'm back at work because I'm not as stressed'…all of these things that come from one person changing. The generations to come and the lack of dysfunction, violence and crime and drugs in the community because of his change, you can't measure that. It's the ripple effect."

ℓℓℓ

Jared's story is a tale of second chances. But for a second chance to take hold, not only does a person need to have the desire for change; The person also needs a support system or organization willing to support them. Willing to send the person letters in jail—even after reoffending. Willing to help the person after he or she backslides into a dangerous lifestyle.

When I asked Jared why he reached out to Live For More during one of the most difficult moments of his life, he said "I could be open and honest. They'd be there no matter how bad I was."

Not only did Live For More support Jared—they did so in a unique way: unconditionally. And that, I learned, is the last remaining aspect that makes their surf therapy organization so successful.

"On paper, if you were to look at Jared's rap sheet, his history, what he's been through as a kid, the amount of time in prison, his age—all of those algorithms the system does—he would be the most high-risk young man that ever came through the doors at Live for More," Krista told me. "Now he's working here. It doesn't make sense. But with unconditional love and support and providing hope for people who are hopeless, anything is possible. Live for More has a faith behind it—we're all Christians. There's a lot of prayer that goes into it, and we see miracles all the time. Our unconditional love for these guys is coming from a place of God's love."

That's the formula for Live For More, a formula that creates stories of second chances, stories of breaking generational cycles of drug abuse and imprisonment. Carefully created programs where participants can experience a feeling of cleansing, a dopamine rush, discover a new identity, and feel unconditional love and support. A lot of prayer, too.

The power of the Live For More story went to even greater inspirational heights with Jared and Krista's marriage in 2021; they have a beautiful daughter who will no doubt grow up surfing. Krista credits their marriage, family, the organization, and their entire story to God.

After I had this answer to how surfing has been therapeutic for Jared and other Live For More participants, I still had one remaining for Krista. The fight to help those behind bars is, like waves on a shoreline, constant, and, as a recent study suggests, more important than ever. Evidence suggests there are more people with mental health and addiction problems in prison today than ever before.

What Live For More has proved is that not only is surfing a form of treatment for young adults trapped in dangerous and deadly generational lifestyles; it is an effective form of treatment.

That leads me to ask this: So, when will it be available to more young adults not just in New Zealand, but worldwide? When will it be available to young adults who, like Jared once was, are behind bars at this moment? They just need someone to believe in them. When will it be available to those who, as Krista said, don't "fall in the cracks" but are "born in the cracks?" When will it be prescribed to those that can benefit from it the most?

"I definitely see it in the future," Krista said. "I don't know how near, but given how quickly surf therapy has progressed even in 4 or 5 years, I'm really hopeful. It's growing exponentially and there's research being done on it, so I think it's a matter of time. You can't deny the evidence. This is working. This is helping. This is saving people's lives. Why wouldn't it be accepted?"

6

SIRENS, PTSD & SURF THERAPY FOR POLICE OFFICERS

At 9:30am, a group of 12 English police officers sit in chairs arranged in a circle inside a two-story beachfront building in Cornwall, located in Southwest England. The officers, dressed in plainclothes, are sitting in silence, thinking about their fears and concerns. They've been handed a piece of paper and a pen and asked to anonymously write whatever comes to mind.

These men and women are protectors, investigators, enforcers. Their workplace involves violence, trauma, or death—sometimes all three in the same day. These badge-wearing individuals are seen as strong, intimidating, almost invincible.

So, surfing with Surfwell—one of the first surf therapy interventions for police and first responders struggling with mental health—should be an afterthought compared to what they experience on the job.

But that isn't the case.

Many of them stare out the tall windows of the historical Bude Surf Life Saving Club towards whitewash crashing on the beach and then begin scribbling.

James Mallows, one of the co-founders of Surfwell, is easily iden-
tifiable with bright blonde hair and is quick to smile. He softly asks
everyone to drop their pieces of paper into a police hat and begins to
pass it around the room. As the hat goes around the circle, he explains
that he'll read off every piece of paper—again, anonymously—to relieve
the fears and concerns of the participants.

When the hat gets back to him, the room still in silence, he picks
the first piece of paper up and reads it off to the group.

"I'm terrified of drowning."

"Well, you won't have to worry about that today, because the
instructor to participant ratio is 1:1, and every instructor here is lifeguard
and water safety trained," James says. "You're all in safe hands today."

With that fear and concern addressed, James takes another piece
of paper out of the hat, unfolds it and reads it off: "I'm worried about
how I'll look in a wetsuit."

After addressing it, he reads off another: "Sharks"; then another:
"I'm worried about becoming emotional or showing emotion"; and
another: "Talking in front of people"; and yet another: "Getting stung
by a jellyfish."

As each fear and concern is addressed, you can see the tension
amongst those in the circle ease; shoulders drop, there's audible exhales,
stiff figures become more flexible, heads nod.

As James explains, the goal of this exercise, and the Surfwell day as
a whole, is to overcome fears, both big and small.

For the participants, overcoming fears started with arriving at
the two-story Bude Surf Life Saving Club an hour or so before this
introduction began. As participants trickled into the car park, Surfwell
instructors James Mallows, Samuel Davies, and others, kept an eye out
for them. The instructors wanted to greet the participants, yes, but they
also wanted to prevent a repeat of a recent incident where a participant
had parked their car, idled, and so fearful of a day focused on mental
health through surfing, drove away.

Once each police officer arrived at the Bude Life Saving Club they were greeted—this time, no one escaped the car park—and entered the room with chairs arranged in circles. James first provided a welcome and congratulations for taking the first step of being present. Then he provided an overview of the day: fears and concerns, a surf session, lunch, a group meeting or debrief, and then a conclusion to the day.

With the fears and concerns complete, the group changed into wetsuits provided by Surfwell and began the walk to the Summerleaze Beach—a right to left breaking wave that wraps into a harbor—about 400 or 500 meters away.

With Sam, James, and other instructors—all of whom are current or former police officers—carrying the large boards, the group exited the building and followed a dirt path up a hill, past a row of colorful beach huts.

Watching from afar, it looks like a group headed for a surf, nothing more. But the reality is much different. These plainclothes police officers face Post Traumatic Stress Disorder (PTSD) along with other mental challenges due to their line of work.

Inside their head, they carry memories of pulling someone out of a mangled vehicle on this side of the road. Memories of being verbally abused, of being physically assaulted, stabbed, shot, informing someone that their loved one has passed away. They remember opening the door to the scene of a murder, investigating child or domestic abuse, and unfortunately, much, much more.

Those of us not familiar with the reality of the emergency services may not realize that all of these situations are experienced just as another person would experience meeting with a client or running business errands. Try switching your 11am meeting with a new client with a police officer being called to the scene of a deadly car crash where both metal and bodies are mangled beyond imagination. Try switching that report your boss wants on his desk by the end of the week with a graphic murder investigation, including photos that you can't unsee. Try switching your work from home day with arriving onto the scene of a fight breaking out—and weapons are being used.

What's more, police officers often go from one of these situations to the next, adrenaline acting as a light switch that constantly remains on, with little to no time to emotionally process what they have seen or experienced.

And on top of that, police officers are there to help the emergency situation—not to be helped. Showing signs of weakness or vulnerability on the job or at home isn't in the cards for them. Because of this, a "macho mentality," where it's not necessarily cool to show or share weakness, prevails. Macho mentality doesn't accept PTSD. Macho mentality doesn't accept mental health as a whole.

Today, some officers came to surf with Surfwell because no other treatment, including the treatment provided by the police force, had helped their PTSD. Some in the group have been treating their loved ones differently and are no longer passionate about what they once were. Others are on the verge of quitting the force completely. And one or two may even be thinking about taking their own life because there seems to be no escape.

This surf session is the last line of defense in the mental battle in the police officer's minds.

Once the group arrives at Summerleaze, the participants staring at the breaking waves with uneasy eyes, James asks everyone to form a circle for a breathing technique to calm the nerves.

James leads them in a 4-7-8 breathing technique—breathing in through your nose to the count of four, holding the breath to the count of seven, exhaling through your mouth to the count of eight—and after some brief yoga poses, beach instruction began. James, Sam, and the other instructors show the participants how to lie on the board, how to paddle, where to place your feet, and finally, how to stand on the board.

Then, the surf session begins: they each walk to the waterline and slowly wade into the sea. For the next two hours, the instructors work with the participant and his or her comfort level. Progress looks different for everyone; some attempt to get into the sea; others try to balance on a surfboard while sitting; some are pushed in whitewash and ride on their bellies; a select few even attempt to stand; others stand and ride the whitewash in.

In between the sound of water rushing by your ears, you can hear cheers. You can hear joy. You can hear excitement.

In each of these actions, whether it's someone simply wading into the sea or someone riding a surfboard towards the sand, something profound happens: the participants begin to open up to the police officer instructors. Phrases like "this is the most fun I've had since an incident on the job" happen. "This feels great!" "I thought about quitting completely." "I thought about taking my own life."

When these conversations start on the surfboard, the healing from PTSD—one of today's most dangerous epidemics amongst police officers and other emergency services—begins.

ℰℰℰ

I discovered that what makes PTSD so dangerous—and so difficult to treat—is that it can be hard to define, and even understand.

Etymology speaking, trauma comes from the Greek word "wound," and post stems from "behind" or "after" in Latin.

The England's National Health Service (NHS) defines PTSD as "an anxiety disorder caused by very stressful, frightening or distressing events."[153]

But that's a 1D look at an issue that, like the brain itself, must be looked at in 3D.

To add more context, I dug through Allan V. Horwitz's *PTSD: A Short History*. "Post traumatic stress disorder is the emblematic mental illness of the early twenty-first century," he writes.[154]

"PTSD indicates a link between a prior negatively valued disruption and some present form of psychic suffering," he continues.[155] That present form of psychic suffering can range from awaking at night and screaming to mental imagery that just won't go away, a sudden avoidance of something that used to be so normal, anxiety, depression, a loss in passion.

PTSD is a subjective disorder in the medical world that diagnoses and treats the objective—and this can change from person to person depending upon age, background, experiences, and cultural norms. Horwitz says:

> *"Personal appraisals of the traumatic quality of events themselves are heavily dependent on collectively held interpretations. Sharp boundaries between traumatic and non-traumatic stressors do not exist in nature. Different cultures draw lines in different places between events that expectably lead to pathological symptoms and those that do not; events that are traumatic in one place or time might be habitual in others."[156]*

Anthropologist Allan Young helps bring the definition of PTSD into 2D by saying that with PTSD, "time runs in the wrong direction, that is, from present back to the past."[157]

To take my understanding of the brain from 2D to 3D, I contacted Dr. Jess Miller. Dr. Miller holds many prestigious titles: Director of Research at Police Care, Principal Investigator at University of Cambridge, and Emergency Responder Consultant for the Royal Foundation. Titles aside, she's an advocate for the mental wellbeing of the police.

"PTSD is phenomenally huge, massively important and completely not dealt with," she told me.

Just how much of an epidemic is PTSD among the police force in England? The answer lies in the sum of two categories: what we can quantify and what we can't quantify.

In her role at Police Care, Dr. Miller ran a study that found that:

- Over 90 percent of police officers and staff were exposed to trauma.
- 1 in 5 live with some kind of PTSD.
- The majority (65 percent) don't feel their force provides adequate support.[158]

But that's only the quantifiable amount of PTSD. There's still an unquantifiable amount that adds even more to these alarming statistics.

Dr. Miller explained that fire, ambulance and police attend to people on some of the worst days of their lives, when they are on the brink of some huge suffering, pain and trauma—daily—and it's hard to quantify that over time.

"It's tricky to put a number on, unfortunately," she said. "It's a very complicated, messy kind of experience in the mind, trauma."

So what we know is that the overwhelming majority of police officers in England are exposed to trauma, with at least 20 percent of the police force actively living with some form of PTSD.

But the true number—the sum of the quantifiable and the unquantifiable—could be far greater.

ꙅꙅꙅ

How does PTSD change your brain?

I asked this question to Dr. Miller, and to provide an answer, she used the hand analogy made famous by Dan Siegel, the clinical professor of psychiatry at the UCLA School of Medicine and the founding co-director of the Mindful Awareness Research Center at UCLA.

She held up her hand and made a fist. She pointed to her fingers, explaining it symbolized the front part of the brain—the prefrontal cortex—pointed to her wrist and explained that it was the brain stem, and then opened her hand and showed that inside represents the command center of the brain—the amygdala and hippocampus. The amygdala is an almond-shaped area that involves emotion; the hippocampus is seahorse shaped and helps us make sense of and contextualize our experiences.

"PTSD's emergence and subsidence lies with the hippocampus," she told me. "It's when the hippocampus fails to make sense of an experience and file it as the past…that is what PTSD is in a nutshell," she said.

The more traumatic experiences you have, like a police officer's daily diet, the more your amygdala fires, releasing stress toxins, which can damage the hippocampus and prevent it from making sense of the event as past and not the present. That's why Allen Young said PTSD is when time runs in the wrong direction. Because the memory isn't filed, it will keep popping up—that's what a PTSD-created flashback is.

"So, they are memories…all of a sudden they aren't memories, they're right in front of your face," Dr. Miller said. "You can see them, but you can't see them. That's all that's about hippocampal functionality."

I asked Dr. Miller if there would be a difference in my brain—someone who hasn't been exposed to the daily diet of trauma—and a police officer.

The answer surprised me.

She explained: "With police officers who have been on the front line or experienced significant chronic stress exposure and haven't learned how to reset and turn off that chemical bombardment of toxins, they are likely to show damage from those toxins on the outer layer of the hippocampus. With people with chronic stress and early exposure to stress, I'd expect to see an underactive, smaller hippocampal area and perhaps an overactive amygdala function..." she paused to note that it's important to factor in changes in the brain due to other life experiences, lifestyles and diet...

"If we're talking about the job and what I know, I would say it would be not unusual and not uncommon to see smaller hippocampus and atrophy there. There are studies that have shown that hippocampi are smaller in police officers who have had trauma and an amygdala that are more active."

The more I talked with Dr. Miller, the more I realized that getting PTSD as a police officer is not a matter of if, but when. So once your amygdala and hippocampus begin showing signs of PTSD and a police officer begins to feel its effects, is there a way out?

"PTSD is not a life sentence," said Dr. Miller. "It's really important not to over-identify with PTSD when you've been diagnosed with it. That's where you fall short. PTSD is a disorder from an incident. And disorder because it's part of your brain that needs to work better. You get your brain working better, it files it away and there's no more disorder."

She continued: "If you enhance and tap into this area of the brain and get it working effectively, any problems in here can be much better resolved. So, if you do have hippocampi atrophy or you are bogged down by trauma and alarm responses, you can do something about it. Without training this part of the brain, you can do very little."

And if you don't address it—if a police officer takes hold of the macho mentality and brushes PTSD aside—complex PTSD can arise, where the trauma becomes even more deeply ingrained.

The police force in England has several ways to treat PTSD. This includes Eye Movement Desensitization and Reprocessing (EMDR) for single incident trauma—typically under six sessions—which uses guided instruction and eye movements to help you reprocess and repair the event that led to PTSD.

Along with that, they recommend trauma focused Cognitive Behavioral Therapy (CBT)—usually 12 sessions—in a clinical setting, and then intensive psychotherapy for Complex PTSD, which can be anywhere from 12–36 sessions or more.

Here's the important question: are these forms of therapy effective?

In her study with Police Care, Dr. Miller found that 65 percent of the police force doesn't believe adequate support is provided.

"A lot of people say I've had CBT, I had the counseling, but it didn't help," Surfwell co-founder Samuel Davies told me. "A lot of police officers will say they have a real barrier with engaging with a counselor because they have this perception that it will be in a clinical setting with an individual who doesn't who doesn't understand what it's like to do the job they do. So how can they advise me? A lot of police officers hold that opinion rightly or wrongly. A lot of people come through desperate for something else to try because they've tried what was available, and it hasn't sorted it out for them."

During a surf session, Sam and James had the same thought on their minds while trading waves: one of their friends in the police force experienced trauma and had been through the counseling, had been through what was offered, but came out the other side no better off.

That's when the lightbulb went off: surf therapy.

eee

Sam and James are typical surfers: dawn patrolling before work, squeezing out a few waves before last light, or filling the lineup during the weekends.

Neither of them could have imagined what that passion would lead to with the police force.

"We experienced a really great surf session after a bad day of work, and both of us said if we could bottle this feeling, it would be amazing," James told me.

This feeling—an ambiguous emotion that so many surfers had felt before, whether it was on their first wave or their hundredth.

For surf therapy to work for police officers, James and Sam knew they would have to prove that it was more than a feeling. They would have to prove hard, quantifiable data that surfing could be therapeutic.

After studying the process and method of surf therapy organizations who had been taking military veterans surfing, James and Sam built a proof of concept that involved surfing, focus groups, and an emphasis on creating a lasting community for the Devon and Cornwall Police.

"Surfwell" was born.

For the pilot program, they partnered with the esteemed University of Exeter, located in Exeter, England, who studied the program from August 2019 to May 2020. The study would include 20 police officers who had been referred to the program by the police force's occupational health team and had current or recent mental health difficulties, graded as mild to moderate in nature.

Each month, a group of two to six officers attended at least one of Surfwell's surf sessions and took part in a pre and post session survey, focus groups, as well as one to one follow up interviews.

The goal of the study was twofold: to measure Surfwell's impact on mental health, wellbeing and performance, and to establish whether surfing is an effective way to confront a wellbeing challenge.

If the study proved that surfing was therapeutic for the Devon and Cornwall police, surf therapy could, in the near future, fill the void where other forms of therapy were falling short.

℮℮℮

Over a year later, Sam and James had been running surf sessions throughout the year during their off time. Demand to surf with Surfwell grew exponentially; it wasn't just signing up; it was joining a waiting list, and sometimes mental health can't sit on a waiting list. Because of preliminary data reports and to meet the growing demand, the police force allowed them to run the program as their day to day job.

Then, the University of Exeter produced a 14-page document that was assuring, thrilling and surprising all at once. "Quick Wins to Long-Term Outcomes: An evaluation of Surfwell for promoting the health and wellbeing of police officers," with a photo of police officer hats in the foreground and a surfboard in the background was 14 groundbreaking pages of reasons why the police force should adopt surfing as therapy.

The data, combined with a demand that continued to increase, allowed Surfwell to expand to eight full time positions, taking dozens of police officers and other first responders experiencing waves of healing each week.

The first part of the study focused on the "immediate gains" police officers experience from going through the Surfwell program, a contrast to, say counseling, which would take session after session before results can be seen.

After a Surfwell event, participants reported an immediate:

- Positive change in mood
- Sense of achievement
- Improved confidence
- Greater acceptance of mental health difficulties
- Renewed motivation[159]

One female participant said in a focus group after surfing:

> *"I'm probably in the worst headspace I've ever been in and I pretty much spent all of Monday crying and so to be here today smiling, is a complete leap…I feel energetic. I feel happy. Like there's this buzz when you come out."*[160]

A buzz. A feeling.

These participants were experiencing exactly what Sam and James felt during their lightbulb moment: an immediate change in how they felt after surfing.

While counseling involved a 1:1 interaction in a white-washed room, the study found that surf therapy offered the chance for participants to interact with peers who were going through similar challenges, which led to another immediate gain—the acceptance of their own mental health issues. One person said:

> *"It's going to be a long standing process in regards to I might never be 100 percent again, if I can put it like that, but [attending Surfwell] was certainly a way in which I gained more perspective of my condition."*[161]

Another immediate gain unique to surfing had to do with body image. One female participant commented:

> *"I always wonder, you know when I put [on] that wetsuit—you can imagine—and I always wonder what other people think and I used to think that for a little while when I was still in uniform and somebody once called me a fat police officer and it really hurt and so, when I went surfing I thought they're just gonna judge me because I've to put a wetsuit on and I'm big and they didn't at all. They just didn't at all and I forgot about my size when I was there."*[162]

In one page, the study had proved that after just one day with Surfwell—fears and concerns, surfing, focus groups, and more—police officers walked out of the sea better.

The goal of surf therapy isn't just immediate gains; it's also sustained gains over time, teaching participants how they can become their own greatest advocate and provide them with self-help tools. The University of Exeter also studied these sustained gains and found that Surfwell enabled participants to develop personal gains that lasted at least 6 to 8 weeks after the intervention.[163]

These personal gains included:

- Growth in resilience
- Growth in hope
- Growth in optimism
- Growth in self-efficacy[164]

Incredibly, five out of nine interviewees reported that Surfwell had helped to reduce their stress levels and created a belief in their ability to cope with their tasks in the coming week. One female participant said:

> *"I've felt so much stress over the last couple of weeks and today I feel better than I've felt in a long time and then I can go back and start again. I'd be like, right let's deal with these challenges."*[165]

What was even more interesting was that six of nine returning participants reported optimism weeks and months after the session—the definition of a sustained gain.[166] It reminded me of parents of children with autism telling me that their son or daughter was different not just for the day, but for weeks after surfing when I was writing *Waves of Healing*.

Another participant said:

> *"It just gave me a sense of being somebody rather than, I'm plodding along every day, getting on, not really getting any answers*

to my problems and my issues, but that I was actually somebody that was worth it—you can't buy that."[167]

Another participant noted that part of the draw to surf therapy is that, well, it is fun compared to other forms of therapy and sports.

"I have other methods of maintaining vague fitness. Walks, cycle rides, things along those lines, but that doesn't give me the adrenaline pure exhilaration that Surfwell does and it doesn't give me that shot of adrenaline/wellbeing that comes from it."[168]

Yes, Surfwell's program could make an immediate difference. It could also make a continued difference in the long term. And as the study examined next, it could have a tremendous effect on the police force as a whole.

ⓔⓔⓔ

Groundbreaking may be an understatement. Positive perception of organizational support, less absenteeism, and higher staff retention— this is how the fears and concerns, surfing, and focus groups, all that makes up the Surfwell program, affected the police force.[169]

As far as positive perception of organizational support, one participant said:

"A project like Surfwell that is clearly intensive in time and money and resources—when you see your own organization commit to a project like that you realize that they are committed to genuinely valuing mental health and wellbeing in the workplace…because often we hear a lot of words and see them clash and that's not the case."[170]

A symptom of PTSD is avoidance, and it makes perfect sense: if a police officer experiences something traumatic on the job, he or she will want to avoid what led to that trauma, and that can lead to prolonged sick leave.

But when a large portion of officers go and stay on sick leave, it can create a dangerous void—other officers asked to work overtime, emergency calls potentially going unanswered.

But Surfwell was able to actually reduce that level of sick leave. One participant said:

> *"From a personal point of view, I've got a lot of things on my mind right now that are not related to work and I know that if I don't have some way to deal with those issues then I'd be off sick quite easily but by doing something like this it keeps you balanced. The organization will gain massively because I'll be at work as opposed to having to backfill me for the next six months."*[170]

Even more impressively, Surfwell directly convinced some officers who had been through traumatic events to stay with the force.

The police force saw a 47 percent increase in the number of UK police officers taking time off with mental health issues from 2012 to 2017—to which the Federation's lead on Police Officer Mental Health said: "There is a systematic failure of care to these officers."[171] But Surfwell was changing that failure.

One Surfwell participant said:

> *"I was on the verge of leaving. I couldn't cope with everything, so I was about to hand in my notice and just say I don't want to do this anymore. I love my job, but I was just struggling at that time, and I can wholeheartedly say the only reason I didn't leave the police was because of Surfwell because of the support*

*I found from the facilitators and peers, 100 percent that's why
I didn't leave the job."*[172]

eee

After examining these groundbreaking results—the immediate gains,
the sustained gains, the organization gains—there was nothing to
debate. James and Sam's crazy idea to take police officers surfing as a
form of therapy was working.

And in the next few years, Surfwell became not only an option for
Devon and Cornwall Police, but for all entire emergency services in
England.

eee

Learning groundbreaking data wasn't the only thing that came from
the study. It was also a chance for James, Sam and the Surfwell team to
learn more about their participants and how they can serve them. Sam
learned a valuable lesson: he can help save a life by simply listening.

"I was chatting with a participant, and the person made a throw-
away comment that they had thoughts that their family and partner
would be better off without her," Sam said. "I picked up on that, and
said 'that's quite a big thing, what you just said.' The person broke
down in tears at that point and we talked over the duration of the day.
The person admitted thoughts of suicide and had gone as far as identifying where in the house it would be done and how it would be done."

Sam realized that this individual needed more professional and
clinical support, and that day became about convincing her to seek
help, and Surfwell referred her to a clinical setting.

"Conversations like those have happened quite a few times," Sam
said. It's eye opening. Before getting engaged in Surfwell, I had no idea

just how common and prevalent these thoughts are among the people in our organization and the wider emergency services in the UK. It's quite surprising."

What also helps create those conversations is that every Surfwell team member is a former or current police officer. Unlike therapists in a clinical setting, those teaching participants how to surf and pushing them into waves knows what they're going through, and, more importantly, has come out the other side of it.

"I think people who come to a Surfwell event know it's helping their mental health, but it gives them an excuse to come because they trick themselves into thinking it's just a surf session, it's just a bit of fun," Sam said. "Counseling is too serious, but this is just a surf lesson because that looks like fun. Once they're there, the overwhelming message is loads of apologies, such as 'I'm really sorry, I don't know why I told you that stuff.' And our response is 'That's the point, it's why we're here. We've been there, we know what you're going through, we understand.'"

"The fact that the instructors are officers is really, really important," said Dr. Miller. "You do need police officers to do it. Because the brain recognizes these people have been through what I've been through. If you don't have police officers doing it, you're on the water having adverse experiences and challenges with someone who doesn't know who you are. Having people who are police trained and police experienced with you side by side to help you get on and off the board and give you a thumbs up when you need it is massive."

ece

As I learned more about Surfwell's story and their impressive data, I marveled at just how unique the marriage of police officers and surfing is—and how rare it is to get to this point.

Surfing's past is that of anti-establishment, draft dodging, a rebellious nature. Police stand for structure, law and order, no rule breaking. Historically, they are two opposing forces, the antithesis of one another that led to citations, middle fingers, sirens and in some cases, handcuffs.

But in the past decade, surfing as a sport and industry has evolved, leaving its past as nothing more than entertaining stories for history books. Surfing is more clean cut, professional, a sport that police officers like Sam and James took up—and now, hundreds more police officers, all for data driven, therapeutic benefits, have done the same.

ℯℯℯ

You can do studies and experiments in a lab all you want, but there's nothing like experiencing your own research for yourself. Dr. Miller participated in a Surfwell event to examine its effects herself and had brilliant takeaways that added more context to the findings from the University of Exeter study.

She saw and felt how the Surfwell environment is, "Great for the prefrontal cortex. It's very fertile ground—well, fertile water."

"There's three elements to the human brain that need to be looked after," she told me. "A sense of safety in the reptilian brain, a sense of satisfaction and reward and having what we need in the mammalian brain, and in the primal brain, the more advanced brain, is connected with others. Surfwell manages to achieve all of those things. It enables safety, connection with others, and shared experiences."

Dr. Miller suggests that surfing can act as a form of EMDR, which is a form of therapy the police force recommends.

"With EMDR, you activate two sides of the brain to get it working more powerfully," she said. "You can do that when you're horizon scanning on a surfboard and you instinctively look side to side, you're stimulating the brain to open up and you're getting a sense of expanse and that whatever brought you to Surfwell that day is in a much bigger pot in this massive ocean in front of you."

She continued: "In British tradition of neuropsychology, we talk about having a strong back and soft front, and I think Surfwell really gives you that because you've got your back to the shore and to what brought you here and you've got this soft opening to this massive ocean and your board and the people around you, which is really, really helpful."

Not only did she see change among others at Surfwell—she experienced the change herself. "I came away from Surfwell feeling a completely different person," she said. "And I'm a neuropsychologist who has practiced mediation and been on two week-long retreats for 10 years. And that afternoon with Surfwell I changed."

Dr. Miller recommends that instead of trying the same form of therapy over and over again with the same unsuccessful result—the definition of insanity—to instead follow the research.

"Go where the science is," she said. "Surfwell creates the model of creativity and engagement with nature, which is really, really important. It creates a model of encouraging the police as an institution to steer away from their traditional thinking, but it also brings fundamental elements of the human brain in terms of engaging with nature and activating the areas of the brain in the right context that we need to do. It's a model for all sorts of interventions that could be based around nature or other environmental conditions."

eee

It's afternoon at the Bude Lifesaving Club. The fears, concerns and anxiety of the morning are long gone; instead, the vibe of the group of 12 plainclothes officers is friendly, warm, and camaraderie fills the room.

Sam told me that at the end of the day, "it's like you're sitting with a different group of people," and he couldn't be more right.

Sam, James and the Surfwell team congratulate the group, and explain how, by taking a day to focus on their mental health, they're different. They look and feel, well, better. And the goal is to take more steps, to keep looking after their mental health, and they can do that through Surfwell's sessions, or by accessing surfboards and wetsuits at specific locations across England thanks to Surfwell and continuing their surfing journey.

The truth is that the participants will return to the difficult job of being a police officer. But this time, they'll have tools and resources that, like a shield, will help protect them now and into the future.

Leaving the Bude Lifesaving Club, seeing the difference in the participants as they return to their jobs, you get the feeling that Surfwell has started something life-changing on the shores of England. And like a wave forming in the sea, it's going to grow.

7

THE SPECTRUM, A BREATH OF LIFE & HOW SURFING HELPS THOSE WITH DISABILITIES

When you survey the populations served across the landscape of surf therapy today, you'll find that most organizations aid those with autism—a broad range of conditions characterized by challenges with social skills, repetitive behaviors, speech and non-verbal communication.[173] It makes sense why as well—it affects 1 in 36 children in the United States, a significantly vast population.[174]

In my previous book, *Waves of Healing: How Surfing is Therapeutic For Children with Autism*, I discovered how surfing was therapeutic for a group of families attending Surfers for Autism events on Florida's coast.

For this book, I was curious to learn more about other autism organizations—including the history behind the original surf camp for children with autism.

I also discovered the fascinating science of how inhaling saltwater vapor when surfing is actually beneficial to participants with Cystic Fibrosis.

What ties both of these populations together is that, through surf therapy, pro surfers treat them to the experience of a lifetime.

ℯℯℯ

Israel "Izzy" Paskowitz was one of nine children. Their father, Stanford M.D. Dorian "Doc" Paskowitz, wanted his family to gain "wisdom that comes from life experience."[175] Instead of living in a house in a cul-de-sac with a white picket fence, they all lived in a camper, "traveling in search of our next wave."[176]

Izzy grew to become a professional surfer, and after marrying his wife, Danielle, they had kids. Their second child, Isaiah, regressed after the age of two and was diagnosed with autism.

One day, Isaiah was having a "meltdown" on the beach at Makaha, found on Oahu's western shores, and Izzy, frustrated but more so concerned about how to help his child, paddled him out into the ocean and saw an immediate change.

> "It wasn't a cure-all for Isaiah, not by any stretch, but for the hour we were in the water, he was a different kid. He was more attuned to his environment. He was laughing and happy. Mostly, he was calm. And for a few hours afterwards he was more manageable, more at peace with himself, and his environment."[177]

After that, it organically grew to taking other kids surfing at San Onofre or Doheny Beach Park.

> "Don't know when or how or why Danielle and I hit on the idea of formalizing what I was doing with these kids. It just

kind of happened, took on its own momentum, and grew and grew. Without really realizing it, without really meaning to, we'd tapped into something bigger than Isaiah…bigger than our own little family…bigger than any of us could have ever imagined."[178]

Izzy was right: it grew bigger than anyone could have imagined. In 1996, Surfers Healing was formed to take children on the autism spectrum surfing—the original surf camp for those with autism. Each year since, thousands have attended their global surf camps, from New Zealand to California, the East Coast, Hawaii, and more.

While some surf therapy organizations push their participants on waves, what makes Surfers Healing unique is they recruit experienced and oftentimes pro surfers—from Zane Aikau, the nephew of Hawaiian waterman Eddie Aikau, big wave surfer Mikey O'Shaughnessy and more—to paddle for the participant and help them ride a wave like an expert so the participant gets to experience the ride of a lifetime.

When I attended events in Waikiki Beach, Oahu and Miami, Florida, I witnessed firsthand as children on the autism spectrum who had never surfed before were suddenly up and riding tandem with pro and experienced surfers, joy wrapped around their faces. And at the end of the day, that's exactly what it's all about for Izzy and the Surfers Healing team.

Izzy writes:

"Sometimes, it was a struggle to get these kids out past the break. In rough surf, I'd have to press them down against the board with my chest, to keep them from slipping off. Some of the kids would be scared; some would be stoked; you could never tell how it would go, but they'd usually calm down once we got on the outside. I'd try to talk to them, if they were verbal; hell, even if they weren't verbal I'd talk to them, because somewhere in there

they were listening. And there was also this; I used to cry all the time for these kids. I'd feel their pain—really feel it. I ached for them, for their parents, for the whole raw deal. But then we'd set about it and for a few moments we'd lift each other from the anguish of autism. We could just surf and hang and have a big old time. "[179]

Because autism rates continue to rapidly increase, there are many organizations in America and worldwide that take children with autism surfing. But Surfers Healing remains unique by providing participants not just with a surfboard, but also a pro surfer to give them a ride they'll never forget.

eee

A morning light casts golden rays onto Ali'i Beach Park in Haleiwa, Hawaii. The beach park is typically crowded on the weekends, but on this Saturday, there seems to be a unique reason for the crowd.

Tents that read "Mauli Ola" sit on the beach, cheers reverberate from the sand as some of surfing's most famous athletes are taking children and young adults surfing. It's a once in a lifetime experience, really—imagine your surf instructor being 11-time Champion Kelly Slater, 3-time World Champion Mick Fanning, 5-time World Champion Carissa Moore, surfing icons like Jamie O'Brien, Kala Alexander, Jack Freestone, Alana Blanchard, and many more.

At first, it's surprising that the participants are going out in the conditions on hand: a 10–15 foot winter swell arrived the night before, and massive waves crash hundreds of yards offshore. But part of the magic of Haleiwa is that these big waves create small waves on the inside of the break—perfect for what's happening.

What's happening on this Saturday morning is surf therapy. The participants each have cystic fibrosis, a genetic disorder that causes problems with breathing and digestion,[180] and, as data has shown, not only is this a fun and unique experience—it helps them breathe better.

eee

In 1999, James Dunlop, along with his brother Charles, two lifelong surfers, started Ambry Genetics, a medical diagnostic company that conducted full gene analysis, and this included stretching DNA to look for disease causing mutations. Clients were asking them to take a look at the genes that caused Cystic Fibrosis (CF).

James didn't know much about it; he soon learned that CF affects about 35,000 people in the United States.[181] After a diagnosis at birth, those with CF have mucus that is too thick and sticky, "which blocks airways and leads to lung damage, traps germs and makes infections more likely, and prevents proteins needed for digestion from reaching the intestines, which decreases the body's ability to absorb nutrients from food."[182]

The goal for every CF patient is to get that sticky mucus out, which can lead to dozens of pills each day, for the course of a lifetime, additional treatments, and hospital stays.

While those with CF are living longer than previous generations thanks to better medical care, an examination showed that in 2019, half of those who had died of CF did so before the age of 32.[183]

The brothers wanted to find a cure for this disease, and in the years to come, Ambry Genetics became "a premier genetics testing lab for mapping the gene mutations responsible for CF."[184]

Around 2007, they discovered an article written in the New England Journal of Medicine, called "A Controlled Trial of Long-Term Inhaled Hypertonic Saline in Patients with Cystic Fibrosis"[185] that talked about the benefits of saltwater for patients with CF.

The study discovered that inhaling saltwater vapor—hypertonic saline—is actually beneficial to patients with CF in their lungs. The

Australian study was inspired by CF patients reporting their lungs felt clearer after surfing and breathing in the fine sea mist kicked up by waves. It was this study that led to the CF treatment of inhaling nebulized hypertonic saline, which is now a medical standard.

With data to support combining their passion with a remedy, James and Charles were sold. They wanted to take patients with CF surfing. After making calls to other foundations and receiving no's—it was too dangerous, they were told—they decided to do it themselves.

They invited six CF patients to Newport Beach to surf. To help teach the participants, they invited pro surfer Jamie O'Brien. Because of Jamie's presence, the surf media outlet Surfline showed up and documented the day and the results. Incredibly, the participants reported feeling better after the surf session. Why was this happening?

It works like this: when the waves crash at the beach, a salty mist is created. Breathing in that salty air lubricates lungs and airways naturally. It also loosens up sticky mucus that is stuck in the lungs. "This makes surfing a natural treatment for anyone with CF which is way more fun than medicine and therapy and hospital visits."[186]

When the article went live, James and Charles began receiving phone calls from parents all over the country asking if they could do the same for their kids. Mauli Ola—native Hawaiian for "Breath of Life"—was born.

The initial challenge with the new organization was preventing cross contamination, something that could be deadly for CF patients. James recalled hearing stories about CF patients being at camps and events in the 1980s, and because their immune system was compromised, they couldn't fight off bacteria that someone without CF wouldn't be affected by. The result, in some cases, was deadly. Because of this, Mauli Ola created strict protocols, which included using anti-bacteria for all equipment, staying 10 feet apart, creating a dirty zone and clean zone, keeping everything meticulously organized.

"Having gone through COVID, now we know what these parents deal with every single day," James told me. "With CF, if your kid gets sick, you don't know if it's the last time he or she will be sick. It's heavy."

With the protocols set in place to ensure the participants were safe from anything bacterial, James wanted to ensure the kids would be physically safe in the water. And the best way to do that was to enlist some of the world's top professional surfers as volunteer surf instructors, from 11-time world champion Kelly Slater to three-time world champion Mick Fanning, surfing legend Mark Occhilupo, Sunny Garcia, Jamie O'Brien, and more.

James recounted, "I would show the parents a picture of one of these guys on a 60-foot wave and tell them your kid is going to be safe in the water with this guy. The goal was to make the parents feel secure and safe."

At each event, whether it's in Haleiwa or another Hawaiian island, California, Texas, or the East Coast, the goal was also to raise awareness for what James calls "the forgotten disease."

While some organizations have to institute time limits to ensure every participant gets a turn, Mauli Ola operates with the motivation that they'll take the participants surfing for as little or as long as they want to.

But Mauli Ola wasn't just putting on surf events. After becoming aware that several CF patients wanted to surf but couldn't leave the hospital, they decided to visit them. Mauli Ola rented a bus, and with pro surfers on board, drove throughout the heartland of America, visiting CF patients as well as other patients in the hospital. "We wanted to do anything that would help raise their spirits," James told me.

In the more than decade since its inception, Mauli Ola has helped thousands of children, and created a tight knit community, including the Labiak family.

Lynn was introduced to Mauli Ola when her daughter, Bree, a CF patient, was about 8 years old. She saw a flyer in South Carolina that offered to take kids with CF surfing to experience fun and therapeutic benefits. After the experience, the Mauli Ola volunteers told Lynn that Bree was a natural. Even better, Bree loved it, and since then, she's traveled and competed at surf contests internationally.

"She could not have picked a better sport," Lynn told me. She explained that, as far as treatment, Bree uses a smart vest. Weighing 13 pounds, it looks like a life preserver. After hooking into a generator, the vest blows up and percusses at certain rates to help break up that excess of mucus. She's done this every day since she was 2.5 years old—and will continue to do it every day of her life.

In addition, there's medicine taken orally. On average, Bree takes 40–50 pills, in addition to aerosol treatments that go directly into her lungs.

"We've never let the immense responsibility of all those medicines and treatments hinder her progress in her surfing because surfing was so healthy for her," Lynn told me. "I'm a true and firm believer that saltwater and surf therapy is an added benefit to everything she already does."

8

SPINAL CORD INJURIES, ADAPTIVE SURFBOARDS & SURF THERAPY FOR THOSE WITH PHYSICAL INJURIES

A t first glance, it's hard to imagine surfing being therapeutic for those with physical disabilities such as spinal cord injuries. After all, for those with movement restrictions, the water can be one of the most dangerous places.

The more I dug into the populations surf therapy can benefit, the more surprised I was—for more than two decades, surf therapy has been helping those with spinal cord injuries, whether it was a condition that someone was born with, or a condition sustained from a traumatic accident.

I discovered a fascinating history behind adaptive surfboards—surfboards that are specially made for those who are restricted in their movement, such as spinal cord conditions—and the incredible work of organizations, instructors, and volunteers to ensure safety. Above all, I realized the lengths that organizations and volunteers will go in order to ensure those with physical disabilities experience the surf therapy.

ⱸⱸⱸ

Staring at the sea in Huntington Beach, California, Jesse Billauer sits in an adaptive wheelchair that is built like a tank. In place of round wheels are triangle pulley systems, which allow the wheelchair to take Jesse onto the sandy beach. Surrounding Jesse is an all-out beach party: tents cover the sand, banners flap in the offshore breeze, loudspeakers blast music, and thousands of footprints are already formed in the golden sand.

Despite this beach party atmosphere, his eyes are focused on the water: directly in front of him, about 20 volunteers stand in the shape of a V while a participant surfs on their belly towards shore. The volunteers are primarily a safety net and secondarily a cheering section, and as the participant rides the power of a crashing wave towards shore, cheers and claps reverberate. Underneath a black hat, a smile forms on Jesse's face.

The events that led Jesse to this moment on the beach—with a smile on his face—have been extraordinary. It began as a story of tragedy, but because of his dedication, commitment, and glass-half-full positive attitude, it became a story of triumph. And a story of life rolling on.

ⱸⱸⱸ

On March 25, 1996, Jesse, along with a few friends, arrived at Zuma Beach in Malibu. It was a weekday, so Jesse, in high school, was in a hurry to get a few waves and get to school on time. Although Jesse often surfed alone, he invited a few friends to come with him this morning. It's this decision that would save his life.

As he slid into his wetsuit on the cold concrete, he could smell the coffee a friend was drinking and could feel the coldness in the air on the California morning. As his feet hit the cold sand, he could feel the light offshore winds, which crafted glassy waves—Jesse paddled out and was quickly up and riding.

By the mid-90's *Surfer Magazine*, regarded as the authoritative "Bible of the Sport," had named him as one of the Top 100 up-and-coming surfers. He was weeks away from turning professional, too. This would be the culmination of hard work and a life's dream. Even better, bigger sponsorships on the horizon meant turning his passion into a profit.

That morning at Zuma Beach, Jesse's talent showed: he caught waves with ease, and produced sharp and spray-infused turns.

Then, the wave that would change the trajectory of his life formed on the horizon. Jesse eyed it and paddled for it. The wave was exactly what he was looking for: it began to suck up and create a dreamy space that he could insert himself into—a barrel. Jesse set his line, and just as he ducked inside the watery tube, the wave throttled him forward. He flew headfirst into a shallow sandbar lurking underneath.

Instantly, he couldn't move. His body floated to the surface, and his back reached air first while his head remained face down in the water. "It felt like someone stabbed me with a fork," Jesse recalled.

It can be terrifying to be in waves struggling to swim, but even more terrifying to be in waves—face down—without the ability to move.

Miraculously, a wave crashed into him and flipped his face skyward; after inhaling, he began yelling for help—to get him to the beach and to keep his head above water.

His best friend, who had just paddled out, towed him back onto shore. "Waves were going over us," Jesse told me. "Saltwater was going in and out of my mouth, out of my eyes, I was hearing a lot of noises. I was nervous. And I was scared."

His friend laid him on the sand—the same cold sand he had just recently walked through. A lifeguard was summoned from a nearby tower, and the first thing he asked Jesse was if he could move.

"I told him that I couldn't move anything," Jesse said.

Jesse remembered the lifeguard cutting his wetsuit off, which Jesse was upset about, because the thick neoprene was expensive—and brand new. There, on the sand, he felt like a "pitchfork" was going through his nervous system. "I felt out of this world, not really there," Jesse said.

As he was placed on a backboard and carried towards the sound of helicopter rotors, his dreams—being a pro surfer, being featured in a surf movie, graduating college—were all flashing through his eyes at once.

"I just couldn't believe the situation."

e e e

In the blink of an eye, Jesse became a part of the spinal cord injury statistics of 54 cases per one million people in the United States, or about 18,000 new SCI cases each year.[187] The estimated number of people with SCI living in the United States is approximately 302,000 persons, with a range from 255,000 to 383,000 persons.[188]

After a battery of tests, doctors informed him that the impact of landing headfirst in the sandbar had broken his sixth vertebrae. He was a quadriplegic, and not only would he never surf again—he would never walk again.

Never walk again?

It was something that Jesse, laying on a rotating bed in the white-light lit room of the hospital with tubes coming out of him, couldn't fathom. He thought he'd be back to normal in a few weeks.

When he was released from the hospital, the biggest challenge of his life began: learning how to live with paralysis.

One of those challenges that Jesse, and those suffering from paralysis, face soon after their initial accident: the cost of medical bills, past and present.

The average annual expenses in the first year after a high tetraplegia spinal cord injury is $1.079 million.[189] And while the costs can vary depending upon the exact diagnosis, the Christopher Reeves Foundation says the expenses don't stop coming. It can cost $75,000 or more each subsequent year.[190] These costs include hospital stays and physical therapy, as well as necessities like wheelchairs and adaptations. For example, a car adaption can cost up to $80,000.[191]

In addition to this, many of those with paralysis suffer the accident early on in life, when they're the most active—which makes it so difficult to grapple with.

I asked Jesse what the hardest part of that shocking change was, and he replied "not being independent. It was devastating to not have independence."

Not only did he need help from family and friends for the big things—groceries, getting fresh air, getting to the bathroom—but also for the small things, like getting the TV remote.

Jesse recalled being at his uncle's house shortly after the accident, where it was just him and a friend. His friend stepped outside, and in doing so, the door locked behind him. Laying in a bed, unable to walk, Jesse didn't know what to do, and the house suddenly felt like a prison. Noticing he was five or six feet from the door, Jesse made a decision. *Let's do this.*

He grabbed pillows and blankets from the bed he was laying on and threw them on the floor. After counting to three, he rolled off the bed, landed on them and crawled to open the door for his friend. This moment gave him confidence that he could accomplish things if he tried.

"After my accident I had a choice," Jesse said. "Was I gonna go down a negative road, stay home, feel sorry for myself and not follow my dreams? Or go down a positive road, still enjoy my life, still follow my dreams. Even though I was paralyzed, that's what I did."[193]

It was set then: Jesse was still going to pursue his dreams with a positive outlook on life.

Jesse, with the help of his brother and their network, started a Foundation called Life Rolls On, which kicked off in 2001. Life Rolls On helps people with paralysis as well as other mobility challenges, including stroke survivors, people born with spina bifida and cerebral palsy and more by holding events nationwide, including in Jesse's home state of California. They Will Surf Again takes athletes surfing, and They Will Skate Again gives athletes the opportunity to skate.

With the Foundation up and running, Jesse wanted to surf again. Along with his friends, former professional surfer Rob Machado and Al Merrick, he worked on an adaptive board that would allow him to lay prone and hold onto the edge—the rails—of the surfboard and steer the board by leaning to the left or right. Once it was designed, they pushed him into the first wave at Cardiff Reef since his accident. The scene was captured in the feature film Step Into Liquid, which was released in 2003.

Even though Jesse was surfing prone, it was still therapeutic. "You feel that rush when you feel that energy," he told me. "The faster I go, the more stoked I'm getting. I'm creating lines on the waves that no one is doing for me. I'm getting to do what I want to do."

Jesse recalled surfing one day and having a profound realization. After getting pushed into a wave by a friend, "I rode a wave all the way to the inside. Floating, I looked up in the sky and I realized all my dreams weren't flashing in front of my eyes anymore. I was living them. I did get to surf in front of 100,000 people at US Open of Surfing in Huntington Beach. I did get to be in a feature film movie. I did graduate college in 2002."[194]

Today, his resume is expansive: aside from his role as Founder and Executive Director at Life Rolls On, he is 3X World Adaptive Surfing Champion, 6X US National Adaptive Surfing Champion, 2X Hawaii Adaptive Surfing Champion, has surfed all around the globe, and continues to inspire others with his message through inspirational speaking.

Where it all comes together is sitting on the beach, in his tank-looking wheelchair, watching others—inspired by his story—surfing.

℮℮℮

Michael Berns was sitting on a surfboard in Malibu in 2008 when he noticed something unusual: within eyesight down the beach, there was a massive event happening—tents, banners, loud music. He noticed people laying flat on surfboards in the water, with about 20 people surrounding them. He paddled in, walked down the beach, and watched his first Life Rolls On event. That day, he signed up as a volunteer, and in 2015 was hired to do Operations for the organization in 2015.

Putting on a Life Rolls On event is a Herculean effort. Michael is in charge of getting equipment to the beach, including wheelchairs, modified surfboards, tents, banners, and flooring they can put down so that the participants—who Life Rolls On calls "athletes"—can access the beach and the shoreline.

Volunteers set up the beach at 6am, with athletes registering by 8am, and the goal is to start surfing at 9am. Each athlete has a color coded "team"—around 20 or 30 people who form a V chute for safety with no holes—"if the athlete falls, the volunteers are there in a second," Michael told me. The team is usually led by a seasoned volunteer, physical therapist, or doctor, and at any time, there can be 300-400 people in the water in total, which does not include the support on land.

There's no doubt: the athletes are putting trust in the volunteers and the organization as a whole, because many of them haven't been in the ocean since their accident, and some have never been in the ocean at all.

That's why it's up to the volunteers to protect them, but also to comfort and encourage them.

"The athletes that come are courageous," Michael told me. "They are putting their lives in other people's hands. It takes a lot of courage to go out in the water knowing one slip up and you can't save yourself—you are in the hands of others. Having the trust of others is an emotional resiliency factor."

Visit the beach on event day, and you'll hear stories of how surfing is therapeutic.

Take Adam Bremen. Born in 1974, Adam was diagnosed with cerebral palsy at the age of two.

> *"I never even thought it was possible for me to surf. Being out here in Southern California, I wanted to give it a shot. Started with Life Rolls On in 2017. I don't know how to swim really, water's cold. All of that dissipated as soon as I got started. It was an incredible day for me, my family and my friends. The freeness and independence the volunteers afford you and the feeling of riding a wave is just epic."[195]*

There's also Ty Duckett, who lost a leg after a motorcycle accident just 15 minutes from where he lived in Southern California.

> *"I thought life was over…My wife had the forethought to find something to replace riding my motorcycle with. She came across Life Rolls On. It gives me that same rush. Before my accident I had never even been surfing. I just knew it looked cool. Didn't think I would ever do it. Couldn't swim and was scared of the*

ocean…It is a rush. It's hard to describe. You can almost liken it to love. Some people have a hard time explaining love. Anything that has you getting up at 5am driving long distances, you have to love that."[196]

Jesse sees the therapeutic aspect on event day as he watches. "When I see the parents of kids who never thought their kid was going to do a sport or surf, I see them cry. There's a lot of emotions. It's a beautiful sight to see, parents crying. It's so much more than just surfing. It's building the athletes' self-esteem. It helps them through the year, become a stronger and more confident person."

I asked Michael how he thought it was therapeutic. "From what I've spoken about with athletes, some love getting in the water, hanging out with us beyond the breaking point, not necessarily catching waves. Some enjoy that emotional cognitive reset. Others enjoy the thrill and exhilaration of catching the wave. With the emotional resiliency factor, it can help in your day to day life outside the water because you have this reservoir of trusting others."

Visit a Life Rolls On event, you'll see Jesse watching with a smile on his face, people thanking him. And you'll see people focused on their ability, not their disability.

ౚౚౚ

Around the same time that Ted Silverberg and his friends were running surf events at Surfrider Beach in the 1990s, a life changing event happened for a man named Danny Cortazzo. It was this life changing event that would put him on the trajectory to helping many—from those with cancer, relatives of those with cancer, quadriplegics and more—through surfing as a form of therapy.

Danny Cortazzo was one of the first Americans to work as a lifeguard in Australia—which provided a great opportunity to surf when not on the clock. But Danny's experience nearly turned deadly. On February 1, 1990, an elderly man lost control of his vehicle and slammed into Danny, who was biking. The collision sent Danny head-first towards a telephone pole. Midair, he miraculously spun around, and his lower back hit the pole. He then ricocheted off the pole, smashed through a fence and rolled down a hill.

A first responder witnessed the terrifying event, and later told the hospital staff that Danny should have been dead, and if not dead, paralyzed.

While recovering, Danny not only realized how lucky he was to be alive—"I had won the lottery ticket," he told me—he also realized how lucky he was to surf. After making a full recovery, he decided to become a paramedic firefighter back in the US to help those who might find themselves in a similar situation. Along with serving as a firefighter, Danny wanted to take those who didn't have the ability to surf on their own into the ocean.

"I realized how fortunate I was to be so connected with the beach and ocean," Danny said. "It also made me aware of how many people will never get the opportunity to experience the joy of feeling the rush of catching a wave. I shared these feelings with my best friends, and we decided to try to help give people with special needs this opportunity."[197]

Along with his four best friends, Danny started the Malibu Board Riders Club in 1992 with several goals in mind, ranging from beach cleanups to fun surf events. Danny's goal was to take kids out surfing who might not ever get that chance. Danny and the Club worked with children dealing with cancer at Ronald McDonald's Camp Good Times.

It was obvious the toll that having a child with cancer takes on the entire family, so Danny took out the family members of those at the house, such as the siblings, surfing. The next day, he took out kids who had cancer, even some who were diagnosed as terminal. He recalled the experience as "amazing."

Years later, in 1998, Danny moved to Santa Cruz, but didn't want to stop taking those in need surfing. That's when he formed Ride A Wave, and what unexpectedly came next was groundbreaking for the organization and for surf therapy equipment in the years to come.

One day, Danny's friend, Sarah Gerhardt—known as the first woman to surf the big wave venue of Mavericks—noticed Brandon in a wheelchair watching waves at the beach with his parents. She mentioned to his parents that it was obvious that he liked to watch the surf. The boy's father responded that he wasn't watching the waves—he was analyzing them. But because of the boy's condition—diagnosed as nonverbal, quadriplegic, and with cerebral palsy—he couldn't get on a surfboard. Sarah connected the family to Danny, who wanted to help him catch his first wave. The issue was how to do so safely.

At a following Ride a Wave event—a cold California day—Danny used a massive 13 foot surfboard and the strength of several volunteers, both at the front and back of the surfboard, to keep Brandon's body on the surfboard and ensure that he could ride waves safely. One volunteer laid stomach first on the front of the surfboard, and Brandon's head was propped up on the volunteer's bottom. Another volunteer sat on the back of the board stomach first as well, helping to paddle and ensure Brandon wouldn't fall off.

After several waves in the cold temperatures, Danny and his team were exhausted, and he wanted to know if Brandon wanted to keep surfing. According to Danny, "I said hey Brandon, look, we're cold and tired, but if you want to go back out, give us a hand paddling and we'll take you back out." Immediately, Brandon's fingers started twitching in the water, and Brandon said "SUUUUUUURF!"

"He did what he could to let us know he was having a blast," Danny said. "It was pretty motivating that Brandon wanted to go back out and keep charging on a freezing and windy day."

"In my opinion, Brandon is a world class surfer, he's just trapped," Danny said. It was this surf session that Danny realized there had to be a more efficient and safer way to take Brandon, and others similar to Brandon, surfing. "I thought there had to be a better way."

With the help of a fellow firefighter, they came up with a design to lock a chair on a surfboard for a participant using air-craft grade aluminum—one of the first known instance in surf therapy of this kind of adaptive equipment being used for therapeutic purposes. From then on, Brandon and others similar to him could utilize these chairs to experience more waves and more of surfing's therapeutic properties in a safe way.

"When you're confined to a wheelchair your whole life, you never experience the thrill that you feel when you're moving fast through the water," Carla Miller, Brandon's mother, told me. "One of his most treasured moments was when he wiped out. A big wave hit him and his volunteers, and he fell into the water. There were so many people around him, so he was picked up really fast, but he loved that unexpected thrill."

According to Carla, the therapeutic benefits extended beyond being in the water. "A lot of the therapeutic aspect for him was the social aspect," she said. "One year, Danny and the organization gave Brandon surfer of the year award. He was known, recognized, and applauded. Another time, I was in charge of pushing his beach wheelchair at an event, and the volunteers were all cheering for him. It's an overwhelmingly wonderful feeling to be cheered like that."

These are multiple instances that may not have happened for Brandon had he not found the surf tribe of Ride A Wave.

The organization worked and continues to work hard to ensure that all participants feel that "overwhelmingly wonderful feeling" Carla alluded to—and, above all, that they feel safe.

Today, during each surf season with Ride a Wave, participants range from children to senior citizens, and volunteers include firefighters, doctors, nurses, EMTs, lifeguards, and more.

Danny echoed the same humble and participant focused mindset that I had heard from others in the sector. "Ride a Wave is not about me," Danny told me. "It's about the people I've surrounded myself with. The volunteers make the program work. There's no way to program what has happened without that support."

9

SURFING PRESCRIBED, MENTAL HEALTH BY STEALTH & SURF THERAPY FOR MENTAL HEALTH

The mental health statistics for two countries in opposite hemispheres is collectively alarming: 1 in 5 Australians have experienced some sort of mental disorder,[198] and one in six people among those aged 6 to 16 in England had a probable mental health condition in 2021.[199]

Instead of continuing down the traditional method of therapy inside four walls, surf therapy practitioners in both countries are taking therapy to the beach—and are seeing tremendous, data driven results with tear-jerking testimonials.

Most of all, their success shows there's hope for a future with positive mental health.

ᴇᴇᴇ

Green and blue rash guards add color to Southwick Beach, located south of London, on a gray weekend morning.

There's nervousness amongst the 20 or so surf participants, ages ranging from 8–17, who are wearing the colorful rash guards: no one is saying much, and a few are still hanging onto their mom or dad's arms. Eyes nervously dart back and forth between the surfboards on the coarse sand and the crashing whitewash rolling in from the English channel.

The next step for the group leaders is to try and calm the nerves of the participants. Led by a surf instructor, everyone sits in a circle and introduces themselves. It's in this circle that the participants are invited to surf, not told to—because at the end of the day, they get to choose what they do today on the beach.

The surf instructor leading the meeting shows the participants how to paddle, how to stand up on a surfboard, and encourages them by describing safety measures—every participant will have a dedicated surf mentor.

After that, warm up games, like crabs and shells, meant to further reduce anxiety, follows. The volunteers act like crabs and if they touch a participant, they become immovable shells. The goal of the game is to be the last crab standing. Yes, it's silly, but in place of tension and silence is talking and laughter.

The surfing follows: for the next few hours, participants, with the help of their surf mentor, catch waves in accordance with their ability. If they want to make sandcastles or swim, they have the freedom to do that as well.

This is what a surf day at a Wave Project, a 6-week surf program spread across 33 locations in the UK, looks like. Incredibly, many of the participants on the beach today at Southwick were prescribed this for mental health challenges.

Among those aged 6 to 16 in England, one in six had a probable mental health condition in 2021,[200] and The Wave Project is on a mission to change this—through surf therapy.

ᥱᥱᥱ

Joe Taylor's first experiences with surf therapy were taking children with disabilities, including autism, surfing in a program called the Freedom Project.

"The participants were so much calmer, laughing and enjoying it," he told me, shocked to see that surfing could have such an impact on a population in need. After seeing this firsthand, he wondered if surfing could be used to benefit more at-risk populations in the UK.

Utilizing his personal contacts with the National Health Service in Cornwall, he had an exploratory meeting in 2010. In that meeting, they decided to see if surfing could help other populations in need—specifically, mental health of children and young adults. The NHS agreed to fund this "pilot scheme." A clinical psychologist was assigned to the program, and if it worked—if it proved to be effective quantitatively—they would provide more funding.

In order to differentiate it from the Freedom Project, Joe called it the Wave Project. Joe had no idea that his organization had just become "the world's first 'surf therapy' course funded by a government health service.

"At the time, I didn't see this as anything long term—I saw it as a short term experiment, really," Joe told me. "I wanted to see if there were benefits to using surfing for mental health."

So, in September 2010, a group of 20 young people sat on the beach at Watergate Bay, Cornwall, for the first Wave Project surfing lesson.

"They had all been diagnosed with mental health disorders, ranging from mild to severe. Some participants had been self-harming, others experienced severe anxiety, low mood or depression. One participant was diagnosed with schizophrenia. Yet to watch them on the beach, none of this was visible."[201]

The first event showed promise, and Joe later saw how powerful it could be with one specific participant.

One participant, named Sam, was diagnosed with selective mutism. Stress and anxiety shut down his capacity, and it had been nearly two years since he had spoken a word.

"During his course, he started speaking again," Joe told me. "We didn't understand the significance really. He was speaking to his surf mentor, asking where to lie on the board, when to pop up. His mind was refocused on what he was doing in the present."

Joe explained that when Sam returned home, he was talking again. "The moment for me was when they turned up to the beach the following week, and they told me the impact it had on him," Joe said. "I was gobsmacked that surfing could have this impact on a young person. I went away thinking how quite amazing it was." The experience was later backed up by the clinical psychologist, and Joe said that that's what drove the growth of the organization: "my desire to see it more… how many kids like this young lad who could be helped by something so simple and so powerful."

"The results of self-evaluation showed that well-being rose among the group overall, with participants feeling calmer, less angry and more connected to each other, after surfing. Young people experiencing anxiety grew in confidence. One young man named Sam, who had a diagnosis of selective mutism, began talking freely again during the course. It was the first time in the UK that surfing had been used to support mental health."[202]

With success found qualitative and quantitatively, the NHS agreed to expand the organization. It grew from Cornwall across the southwest of England to North Yorkshire, Scotland, Wales, Northern Ireland and even London, where they began taking children from the city concrete onto the sand at Southwick Beach and putting them in colorful rashguards.

Now, sessions are delivered on both the weekdays and weekends, in accordance with the program and the participants schedules, and the Wave Project provides transportation, because without it, many wouldn't be able to attend. This helps to make the surf therapy program available for all despite social or economic barriers.

The Duke and Duchess of Cambridge even visited the organization in September 2016. With William wearing a blue suede jacket, and Kate standing out in a pink dress, they spent more than an hour on the beach in Towan Beach in Newquay, hearing testimonials as huge crowds looked on.

Between 2013-2017, the number of people referred to The Wave Project more than quadrupled, from 100 in 2013 to 461 in 2017. Even though the initial data was promising, further data solidified its effectiveness:

> *"Over three iterative phases spanning five years (2013-2017), a UK-wide surf therapy evaluation program has developed in collaboration with clients, parents/carers, volunteers, referrers and staff. By conducting a programme evaluation that adheres to professionally accepted standards of practice, the Wave Project has been able to empirically demonstrate a sustained, positive impact of surfing on vulnerable young people's wellbeing over time."*[203]

The same study also discussed this empirical evidence more specifically:

> "Participants show transformation in their lives, shifting from isolation to engagement with others through a combination of surfing, volunteering, and mentoring. Clients and their families describe great benefit from this shift and their stories about themselves and their real lived experiences become markedly different. Further unfolding of these stories will be valuable for practitioners, policy makers and academics seeking to understand the health and wellbeing benefits associated with surf therapy."[204]

On top of that, data showed that it had an effect outside the water—both at home and at school.

> "The intervention resulted in a significant and sustained increase in wellbeing. One year later, 70 percent of clients regularly attend a surf club and many have become trained as session volunteers. Parents and referrers noticed an increase in positive attitude and better communication, as well as improved self-management and behavior at both home and school. It is concluded that the Wave Project provides a demonstrable and cost-effective way to deliver mental health care."[205]

The Wave Project also showed that it can help participants long into the future. A transformation narrative emerged which is illustrated by the following account from the mother of Harry, aged 13, who had been referred to The Wave Project:

> "[He] had been excluded from school, didn't really have friends, wasn't part of any clubs. This wasn't for the want of trying, he just didn't fit in, he couldn't follow instructions therefore

it would end with yet another negative experience. He didn't really see anyone apart from immediate family. I could see my boy becoming more withdrawn. The [Wave Project] lady on the phone put me at ease and told me he would have fun so we signed up … He is back in school now, he has a few buddies and he has stuff going on in his life… The Wave Project was very important at a time when he needed it and he will always be a part of it. He now goes to other activities, but we would have been reluctant to try these before. He had a foundation because he succeeded at the Wave Project first. "[206]

Because the Wave Project has been backed by the NHS since its inception, studying the effectiveness of surf therapy became as routine as the surf lessons themselves. The result? A treasure trove of evidence-based data to pull from.

In 2021, they delivered surf therapy to more than 800 participants. Using pre and post surveys from students, participants recorded their wellbeing before and after a course based on a five point scale.

They found:

- 11.63 percent increase in calmness
- 12.2 percent increase in resilience
- 14.9 percent increase in confidence
- 10.3 percent increase improvement in friendships
- 5.6 percent increase in social trust[207]

The Wave Project was also one of the few national UK charities that maintained a full service throughout the COVID Pandemic of 2020, as the country experienced three lockdowns. 16-year-old Dylan, who struggled with low motivation and fatigue, did the program and after just three sessions, he was getting up at 7am. "The Wave Project was a lifeline in lockdown,"[208] his mom said.

"The Wave Project provides therapeutic intervention in the least clinical way possible," said Dr. Alex George, UK Youth Mental Health Ambassador.[209]

ⓔⓔⓔ

What makes the Wave Project so unique is that, as of 2023, it continues to be the only government funded surf therapy program in the world.

So how does it work?

Joe explained the short way for it to happen: in Cornwall, a young person can see their General Practitioner. The General Practitioner can make a referral to the Wave Project, and the organization can support them. Plus, it's free for that person.

Though, there are caveats: Joe explained that if you went to Wales or Scotland, it wouldn't be available in the same way. "It's not available everywhere," he said.

Joe also explained another way that, although it takes more time, the referral result is the same. "Patients would say 'I'm feeling down' or 'depressed, I don't want to go into school. I don't think anyone likes me.' The normal procedure is that the doctor would ask them to fill out a standard survey, a PHQ9." That survey would then be used to make an assessment whether or not they're depressed. "The patient might get a referral to a child psychiatrist, who would diagnose a condition, and refer him or her to surf therapy. A doctor who knows surf therapy might shortcut all that."

"They were encouraged to think about ways they could innovate and look at longer term health problems they were trying to solve," Joe told me, looking back on the original meeting in Cornwall that saw the creation of the Wave Project.

"The funding came out of that thinking … If we support this charity, then it could save us money longer term. And there's no doubt, for the people we worked with, it has saved money. It's improved mental health and there's been less engagement with other health services."

Joe did say that as the Wave Project developed, "the NHS moved away from that thinking; they're more of a reactive service today."

Therein lies the key: being a proactive service. Surfing may not be a one size fits all cure, but by "getting people at risk of mental health issues to start thinking more positively about life about surfing, it might help it avoid bigger problems later."

Joe said, "I feel that we've opened the door to this but not necessarily grasped the opportunity. There have been GPs here in the UK, first point of contact for most things, support it and refer to it but not all of them do. One of my challenges is trying to persuade the NHS more broadly."

Not only does the Wave Project conduct surf therapy; they also raise awareness for doctors to receive more referrals.

Joe likened surf therapy to a recent evidence based practice that has taken the UK by storm: cold water swimming.

"When I started the Wave Project, cold water swimming was very niche," Joe told me. "Now everyone does it. Research came out to show that it's something anyone can do. Go and jump in the lake. Surfing is difficult to organize. As that evidence grows, that infrastructure will follow."

On top of that, Joe sees it growing. "Let's be prepared for when that change comes. It's only a matter of time when it's recognized. There's something about surfing that's quite unique and has really meaningful health benefits for people. I don't think people believe it yet, that's the problem. When it is recognized, I think that change will happen quickly. I think surfing will become much more about health and well-being. Ordinary people on the street will do. Good to reduce your anxiety."

"It's a slow burn now," he said. "But there will be a big bang at some point."

On the other side of the globe from Joe Taylor, the Royals, and the Wave Project, Australia—the land down under—is facing a similar dilemma surrounding mental health struggles: the Australian Bureau of Statistics (ABS) reported that around one in five Australian adults have experienced some sort of mental disorder.[210] When you factor in Australia's population, that's around 5 million people.

The statistics are even more staggering when you turn the spotlight on young adults, those ages 4-17.

One study explained:

- 1 in 7 young Australians ages 4-17 experience a mental health condition in any given year, while 13.9 percent of children and young people meet criteria for a diagnosis of a mental health disorder.
- 1 in 10 young Australians ages 12-17 engage in self-harm, 1 in 13 will seriously consider a suicide attempt, and 1 in 40 will attempt suicide. Suicide continues to be the biggest killer of young Australians.
- What makes helping this populations so difficult is that young adults are less likely than any other age group to seek professional mental health help or support.[211]

One organization is using surfing to address the massive need—utilizing a "mental health by stealth" method that doesn't feel like therapy—and is seeing evidence-based, life-altering results.

ꙮ ꙮ ꙮ

Joel Pilgrim, who surfs 1 foot and 20 feet waves with the same youthful exuberance—and has been doing so for more than two decades—worked at The Bondi Community Mental Health Centre in New South Wales as an Occupational Therapist, serving in the early psychosis community outpatient service.

One of Joel's biggest conversation points is that we're constantly working on our physical health—exercising, dieting, our physical appearance—but not realizing we need to be doing the same with our mental health.

At The Bondi Community Mental Health Centre, Joel witnessed firsthand the limitations of therapy inside 4 walls. "I was seeing just how closed-off people were when talking about their mental health," he told me. "They were unable to share their challenges, and therefore unable to download or debrief. I saw how it was having a detrimental impact on their recovery."

Joel wanted to do whatever it took to help his clients achieve their goals, and this was tested when one client wanted to surf. The client had surfed in the past but had put on weight as a side effect of antipsychotic medication.

"I took it upon myself to provide that opportunity for him," Joel told me. "I could have gotten in a lot of trouble taking this clinical risk." But it was Joel's job to get him back to positive mental health—and it was a risk Joel was willing to take.

They paddled out at Maroubra Beach in South Sydney. "It was almost as if he was a totally different person," Joel said with emotion in his voice. "He let his guard down, and we connected in a laid back way, without the clinical setting, without me sitting across from him in a chair asking to share his experiences."

It became evident that the outdoors was a far more effective setting to connect and explore the intricate concepts of recovery—rather than the traditional clinical setting he had been working in.[212]

"That was a pivotal moment for me," Joel said. "I realized we have to create this opportunity for more people. If this is what's possible for one person, imagine what we can do for groups of people around Australia!"

Though the idea for a surf therapy program was planted, it took time and endured trials before bearing fruit.

"Over six months, I drew up this 50-page manual, and submitted it to the head of mental health in Sydney," Joel said. "And she said that I've got rocks in my head. She said, 'You're dreaming!'"[213]

In the surfing euphemism, Joel kept paddling out even though waves were pushing him backwards towards shore. Eventually, he made it past the break and paddled into the wave of his life—The Waves of Wellness (WOW) Foundation.

Using trained mental health professionals as surf coaches, the organization delivers innovative mental health support programs.[214]

"For many, surfing is an Australian rite of passage," Joel said. "It's a mainstream activity which a lot of the population either observe or aspire to do. We allow people an experience they wouldn't necessarily get if they're unwell."

Joel mentioned that, in Australia and around the world, mental health is a "taboo topic." Combining it with surfing has a powerful effect: it draws it out of the darkness and helps build skills for managing your own mental health.

Since its establishment in 2016, WOW has developed and delivered high-quality programs across a range of demographics; men's health, veterans, first responders, post-traumatic stress disorder, disaster relief, youth, trauma, disability, grief and loss, indigenous, refugees and women's programs.[215] As of August 2023, the organization has run over 362 programs, reaching more than 3,868 participants with over 18,928 instances of participation.[216]

What makes WOW unique is that they have several "surf experience programs"—all of which feature Cognitive Behavioral Therapy (CBT)-based mental health discussion topics that help participants improve their mental fitness.[217]

These sessions are facilitated by surf instructors who are also WOW mental health clinicians, and a 1.5-h surfing lesson follows each discussion.

The study "*A grounded theory exploration of programme theory within waves of wellness surf therapy intervention*," authored by Jamie Marshall published in *Psychology and Health* in 2023, interviewed WOW participants, and discovered five therapeutic categories that are foundational to WOW program theory—and show the evidence behind their therapy programs.

The first category was "Safe Spaces." It's clear that participants experience benefits from the organization and the instructors alike creating a judgment free zone on the sand and in the water. One participant said:

> "*They would talk about like, semi personal experience or like things that they've been through which, which was like comforting in the sense that like when you go to a psychologist, you don't get that personal, whereas the WOW guys were like, you know, I, you know, went through this, like they wouldn't go into like a lot of depth or anything but it made it feel more like a conversation and like a friendship group rather than like a psychologists office.*"[218]

This speaks to the "mental health by stealth" method. In a country where young adults are the least likely age group to seek therapy, WOW doesn't force them into therapy—they provide them a unique experience and open up the floor for them to talk—both of which are stealth therapy measures.

The same study found "This combination of removing judgement, participant-determined pacing and participatory approach to facilitation seem to have allowed for 'mental health by stealth,' avoiding perceived negative power structures and stigma associated with some traditional support settings."

Another participant summarized all of this: "By the end of it, it honestly felt like I'm meeting up with a group of friends rather than going to a therapy session."[219]

Joel explained that some of their surf programs simulate a hospital ward treatment but takes away the hospital. "We do it in a way that doesn't bring the stigma, and it's fun and accessible to people," Joel said. "I call it health by stealth. People are able to learn how they can manage their own mental health."

The second category foundational to WOW's success that emerged is "Social Support." By meeting other participants facing similar struggles, the group not only discovered common bonds that reduced the daunting feelings of isolation—by sharing in the act of surfing, camaraderie was born. One participant said:

> *"We all share each other's success, like, whether it be like, you even just paddled out to get out of the back, which was an enormous task for me and like some other people, that was like a sense of, like, success for the whole entire group. So, it wasn't like individual success. It was success together."[220]*

Another participant said:

> *"It makes you really happy because you're part of a group and you've got people watching and cheering you on. It's like a little like when they say you've got cheerleaders cheering you on."[221]*

Just by being in that group setting—not necessarily talking, but listening—can be therapeutic, something another participant experienced firsthand. This participant's father died by suicide, and although he felt waves of grief, he joined WOW's program. Dave Kelly, a Lead Facilitator with WOW, talked about how powerful the experience had been for a participant.

> *"A participant came down from the hospital. Brought down by a clinician and participated in a group. The parent died and*

he became quite unwell as a result of being depressed and the loss of his parents. He didn't do much talking but he did a lot of listening and a lot of surfing. He was experiencing a lot of joy and being engaged in a group of people. Twelve months later I ran into him at the University and he had gone through some recovery. He was looking really well. Seeing him so well, for me, was more success than I had seen than 10 years of mental health nursing. Because it was such a rapid and positive recovery."

Another category that emerged is "Sensory Grounding." The texture of the sand, the crashing of the waves, the wind on your face…all provided feelings of being grounded in nature. One participant said:

"I feel like it takes away awkward silence because there's more going on. You're not just in like that kind of sterile room and just like, waiting for someone to talk. I feel like silence in nature isn't awkward […] it just isn't awkward because there's more going on. And I feel like it's probably also like it just kind of helps you think and reflect because there's like a bit of silence, but it's just like engaging your senses. It's not a distraction. Just kind of helps the focus."[222]

The fourth category that emerged was "Mastery." Sitting, laying or standing on an unstable surfboard can be a challenge itself—and adding wave riding to the mix can seem like the ultimate test of skill. Succeeding in any aspect of it can lead to a tremendous sense of accomplishment, and deservedly so.

One participant said:

"When you're surfing, and like I stood up quite a few times, like feeling like you accomplished something, like, that was really an important feeling in that process. Because I don't

think when you go through traditional forms of therapy like you're feeling like tangible benefits or tangible things you feel like you've accomplished. A lot of it is like, deficit talk, like you know, I struggle with this. But with your surfing you're actually achieving things."223

The last category that emerged was "Respite"—participants felt they could escape from negative thoughts or mental health symptoms through the act of surfing.224 One participant said:

"A lot of the time, you talked about something very dark or very heavy or something that had weighed on your mind. And as I said, I think surfing is something that people can get a lot of clarity, and like mindfulness out of because really, when you're trying to get a wave and when you're on a wave, that's what you have to focus on. So, I think it's a good way like kind of getting refreshed and processing everything you've just discussed."225

One young participant keyed in on the respite aspect of surfing by explaining how their parent had self-harmed and died. As a result, the young participants wanted to do the same. But surfing "sucked all the bad feelings away."

The last two categories that emerged—Mastery and Respite—speak to the inherent therapeutic properties that all surfers and adrenaline seekers experience: flow state.

In the groundbreaking book *Flow: The Psychology of the Optimal Experience, Mihaly Csikszentmihalyi* defines flow as an "optimal state of consciousness" where we are completely immersed and focused on the task at hand, we perform our best, and, on top of it all, we feel the best.226

Flow isn't something you wake up and step into; it's something that you make happen, by, for example, going out of your comfort zone and signing up to surf with the Waves of Wellness Foundation.

> *"The best moments usually occur when a person's body or mind is stretched to its limits in a voluntary effort to accomplish something difficult and worthwhile. Optimal experience is thus something we make happen."*[227]

As Csikszentmihalyi explains, getting into flow isn't something that is done easily—like attempting to make it past the breaking waves for the first time.

> *"Such experiences are not necessarily pleasant at the time they occur. The swimmer's muscles might have ached during his most memorable race, his lungs might have felt like exploding, and he might have been dizzy with fatigue—yet these could have been the best moments of his life. Getting control of life is never easy, and sometimes it can be definitely painful. But in the long run optimal experiences add up to a sense of mastery-or perhaps better, a sense of participation in determining the content of life—that comes as close to what is usually meant by happiness as anything else we can conceivable imagine."*[228]

Or, as Steven Kotler explains in the *Art of Impossible: A Peak Performance Primer*, the neurobiology of flow is the mechanism beneath the art of impossible.[229]

For participants with WOW, flow can be the conduit to surfing, and, more importantly, healing.

What I found interesting about WOW's programs is that they don't just take participants surfing for weeks at a time—they provide tools for them to continue their mental health fitness journey beyond the program. They do this through surf schools with discounted surfing lessons, discounted surfboards, and wetsuits from industry partners. That, plus participants are also connected via WhatsApp upon completion of their program and continue to meet outside of formal WOW programming.[230]

Joel summed up the WOW ethos by saying: "We're finding people coming to us from so many different places saying, 'there's no way I would access mental health support, but we're coming down to surf therapy'—hell yeah!"

10

WAVE POOLS, INLAND SURFING & THE FUTURE OF SURF THERAPY

While making any sort of prediction for the future of surf therapy—and the future itself—would be unwise, there are hints at what the future of it could look like in the coming years and decades with the confluence of two powerful elements: surf therapy and wave pool technology.

A large part of what makes the sport of surfing—and surf therapy—exclusive is its location. For example, here in the US, almost 40 percent of the population lives near the sea,[231] with the majority of the population living inland. And for this majority of Americans, only a select percentage have the means to travel to the sea and buy or rent surfboards.

If you could somehow bring the waves to those inland, the problem would be addressed. While we don't have magic wands, we do have wave pools.

But before we talk about the possibilities of wave pools, we have to acknowledge their complex past that's rife with unmet promises—and financial failure.

Acquiring land, building a pool, and developing the technology to generate a wave—just for a business to open its doors—has proven to be challenging. A wave pool keeping its doors open has proved to be equally challenging.

Interestingly, the idea of a pool churning out waves has been around for longer than you'd expect. In the 1870s—yes, more than 150 years ago—King Ludwig II of Bavaria installed an electric wave machine in a man-made underground lake at his Linderhof Palace.[232] London's Wembley Swimming Pool, a paddle churning prototype, opened in 1934,[233] and as far as America's exploration into the market, it began with Big Surf, a wave pool located in the last place you'd expect—the middle of the Arizona desert—that was powered by a three story, seventy thousand gallon rectangular cistern, opened in 1969.[234] Wave pools even crowned a world champion: Reigning World Champion Tom Carroll beat future world champion Derek Ho in the finals in the 1985 World Inland Surfing Championships held at, again, the last place you'd expect—Wildwater Kingdom in Allentown, Pennsylvania.[235] In the 1990s and 2000s, wave pools continued to sprout up here and there, but the truth is that none of these were built just for surfers; instead, surfing was part of the adventure experience.

This was supposed to change with the Ron Jon Surf Park. Slated to open in 2005, it was a $10 million dollar "Surfpark," which included three wave pools in Orlando. It was marketed as the surfer's dream, but when it had a soft opening in 2006 and the public saw that the waves were barely surfable, it was hard to imagine someone paying hard earned cash to surf such a terrible wave. When the Recession hit in 2008, the project was scrapped completely.

One wave pool that has lasted the test of time is not far from the failed Ron Jon Surf Park. Inside Walt Disney's World's Typhoon Lagoon, you'll find waterslides, a lazy river, and a massive wave pool—which during certain evening hours, offers chest high surf.

In 2014, I surfed the wave pool for myself. I was surprised at the size of the wave—I had expected something barely catchable and was thrilled to be going down the line. In an article for Eastern Surf Magazine, I wrote about how the wave pool experience was less about the quality of the wave and more about the act of simply surfing:

> *"During long flat spells, we East Coast surfers no longer feel that burning desire that gets us up at 5:00 am to check our local spot on a cold winter morning. We don't feel the sheer joy that comes with seeing an outside set lining the horizon. But wave pools can light that fire that we only feel when we surf. They have the potential to remind us why we love the things we love."*

That's all I thought of it at the time—a reminder of how fun surfing in the ocean can be during flat spells.

But since then, thanks to a "wave pool arms race," it has become much more. Wave pool dreamers have learned from the mistakes of the industries' forefathers, and enthusiasts set out to make more affordable ways to create wave pools, reach different industry sectors, and deliver on the quality of the wave.

Based in the Basque Country near San Sebastián, in northern Spain, the Wavegarden built its first "wave garden" prototypes in 2005, and pro surfers tested them around 2010-2011. It was a unique take on the wave pool template: instead of massive pools costing millions of dollars, the Wavegarden technology was small, quiet and, best of all, produced a surfable, attraction-worthy wave. Because of this successful business model, in the years to come, Wavegarden wave pools would soon open their doors to surfers in Brazil, Australia, South Korea, Switzerland and other locations.

Of course, in 2015, Kelly's Slater's Wave Ranch—the same pool that participants in MeWater surfed in—redefined surfer's expectations. From that point on, when surfers thought of wave pools, they no longer thought about the failures of old; instead, they were excited about the technology and curious to give it a test.

Now that we understand the context of wave pools, past and present, it's impressive that one inland pool destination in Bristol, England, is not only meeting expectations for surfable waves and a unique surfing experience: it's changing lives through surf therapy.

ecc

Nick Hounsfeld, a life-long English surfer, was treating people of all ages, backgrounds and abilities as an Osteopath. But he felt like he wasn't making enough of an impact.

"Suddenly, I wasn't feeling fulfilled with what I was doing at the time," Nick told me. "I was very limited in the impact I could create."

Nick wondered how he could improve people's health and well-being in a completely different and unique way. He wondered: "How can I create a different narrative that is more engaging, more marketable, and combine it with surfing, water and waves?"

Then, he saw footage on YouTube from a Spanish company called Wavegarden, that had managed to create perfect surfing waves on a lake, inland. It was his eureka moment. He soon visited the Basque country to learn more about the prototype, and after that he was all in.

When he spoke with friends, family, and investors to financially back the idea around 2010, he received the same reaction: "Oh, well… that's bonkers! But…you definitely have to do it!"

Even more challenging, Nick wasn't a traditional businessman. He wasn't an investor. However, seeing the potential, and being driven by a strong sense of purpose, he was going to see it. "It didn't matter how long it took, or how hard it was going to be. We just had to do it."

There were several challenges, one of them being not only finding land, but the right land. Nick explained that he wanted to find a beautiful and picturesque area to combine "green space and blue space together."

The Wave opened its doors in 2019, and since then, has become a premier English surfing destination, inland. If you choose a day trip, you can walk through its sliding glass doors, following a sign that reads "All Surfers This Way," and you'll find an aesthetically pleasing surf shop and in a separate area, a cafe with mouth-watering food options. You can even spend the night next to the waves in a camp, which is organized in sections named after surf breaks around the country.

Then, there's the wave itself. From above, it looks like a massive triangle, but the bottom of the triangle is bent outwards. There are two halves to the surfing lake, with a pier separating them. The more advanced surfers catch waves in the Reef area, at the tip of the triangle, whilst beginners learn the ropes in the whitewater waves of the Bay area. In 2022, the Wave delivered 148.5K hours of surfing, welcomed 40K paying spectators, and had 1,218 stays at The Camp.[236]

But The Wave isn't just for surfers seeking a thrill, it's about bringing the power of water and waves to all and has also become somewhat of a hub for surf therapy—and they've been incredibly busy with this!

In 2022, The Wave:

- Supported 122 adaptive surfers.
- Ran four 6-week surf therapy courses with The Wave Project, alongside a regular Surf Club for children that have been through a surf therapy course previously.
- Worked with their partner Dryrobe to provide additional adaptive surfing equipment, such as prone boards.

- Hosted the English Adaptive Surfing Open for the third time, which included Over 40 athletes from around the globe.
- Collaborated with I Am Possible Foundation and Koalaa Prosthetics to develop and launch a 'surf tool' for those with upper body limb differences that helps with popping up to stand on a surfboard.[237]

In 2021, The Wave ran four 6 week surf therapy courses in partnership with the Wave Project—the same organization that sees surfing prescribed—for populations who struggled with physical and mental health issues, social deprivation or social isolation. One parent watching their child said:

> *"I saw him smiling in what felt like the first time in two years, standing on a board surfing towards me. I don't think he's felt pure joy in all that time. The world inside his head is a pretty dark place. This got him back into simple reality. It's priceless."[238]*

One of the main questions surrounding wave pools is how different they are from surfing in the ocean—and whether that's an advantage or disadvantage. So, I asked Nick how it differed.

"Not massively," he said. "You wouldn't notice a huge difference."

He did say there was a difference in the color of the water: "It's much bluer than the ocean here in the UK." And it's a much safer environment, given there are lifeguards constantly monitoring, there are no rip currents, and the waves can be turned off at the push of a button if there's an emergency.

The biggest advantage of a wave pool is the consistency of waves. "We have the ability to consistently produce waves at the push of a button…there's comparable waves only about 30 percent of the time in the UK," Nick told me.

Even though it's not a normal ocean environment, there's still the sound of waves, the sound of people having fun. "The more and more people experience it, they come back to us and say it was one of the best days I've ever had and it reset my body physically and mentally," Nick said.

"I refer to wave pools as health and wellness centers," Kris Primacio, CEO of the International Surf Therapy Organization, told me. "For individuals unable to access oceans, lakes, or rivers, wave pools can serve as a valuable resource for surf therapy."

According to Nick, there's a massive need for inland surfing for therapeutic purposes. "I feel the need is way bigger than what anybody thinks," he said. "We know that when people have a surf therapy intervention down by the sea, how important that is for them, and how truly transformative it can be. So many people in landlocked areas don't even know how incredible that can be. There's loads of people, millions of people, based in UK cities who don't know how good it can be. Wouldn't it be amazing to be able to give more people that taste of the ocean and surf therapy for the first time?"

This hints as to what surf therapy could look like in the future—conducted in the ocean, of course, but also, inland.

"I don't think people understand it yet…I'm hellbent on people getting access to it," Nick said.

eee

"As of this writing, there are dozens of wave pools under construction around the globe, all of which aim to bring surfing inland—but one wave pool stands out because of its commitment to surf therapy, even before breaking ground. Plus, it's the only pension fund backed wave pool to date."

Lost Shore Surf Resort, set to open in 2024 just outside of Edinburgh, Scotland, is expected to become a global tourism destination—a 60 acre country park[239] including a Wavegarden-fueled wave pool, a waterfront restaurant, food market, surf school—and an emphasis on surf therapy.

Edinburgh Napier University created a new research group in partnership with the company to explore several aspects of surfing—high-performance surfing (including Olympic pathways), disability surfing, and equipment research and development[240]—and surf therapy.

The partnership, which will be called Surf Lab, represents a global first in terms of a formal research relationship between further education and a wave pool.[241]

"If we try and replicate the surf therapy experience on the perfect day from the ocean, that's the wrong way to approach it," Andy Hadden, the founder of Tartan Leisure Ltd, who is spearheading the £55m effort, told me. "Wave pools can be a slightly different type of surf therapy experience, so it doesn't feel like you're getting therapy, a health by stealth approach as it were. We also have the opportunity to tailor sessions to participants' needs with predictability and structure unique to the wave pool setting. We want to use this controllable nature of our pool to explore, understand, and maximize our ability to help as many people as we can, which is where the Surf Lab comes in."

Dr. Jamie Marshall, who was funded by the Lost Shore Surf Resort as he undertook the first ever Surf Therapy PhD, sees the wave pool—and the university partnership—as something that will grow the sector to great heights.

"The Surf Lab collaboration is hugely exciting, not just for Lost Shore and Edinburgh Napier University, but for the whole surf therapy sector," Jamie told me. "For the first time in the world, we have a surf specific research group being given unparalleled access to a wave pool location with huge implication for the kind of research questions we can now ask. The controllable elements of the pool enable replication and consistency within studies, allowing us to go deeper into specific elements of the surfing experience whether high performance, leisure based, or therapeutic in nature. I can't wait to see the research outputs that will emerge from the Surf Lab over the coming years."

℮℮℮

In my experience, it's clear that wave pools will never replace surfing in the ocean, but they can certainly supplement the experience. Best of all, as Kris Primacio alluded to, they can serve as mental health centers for future generations—and further open access to surf therapy for those who otherwise couldn't experience it.

FINAL WORDS

After putting the finishing touches on this book, I shut my computer, grabbed my surfboard and boardshorts, and hurried out the door.

While working on *Surf Therapy*, I said "no" to more surf sessions than I would have liked to, and with clean, baby-blue water lines breaking left and right just miles down the road, I wanted to make up for the lost time.

Once at the beach, I waxed my surfboard with wax I'd discovered in the back pocket of my boardshorts, stretched, and quickly paddled out to the lineup. Moments later, a set rose above the horizon, and after letting a few other surfers go, I took the last wave: a long and crumbly blue water left shot me forward. I held my line as the wave reformed on the shallow sandbar and accelerated me all the way to the beach.

As I paddled back out, I couldn't help but think of what was happening based on what I had learned when writing *Surf Therapy*. A safe yet addicting level of dopamine had flooded my limbic system— and produced the smile on my face—as I made my way back to the lineup.

Waiting for another set to come through, I couldn't help but reflect on *Surf Therapy*. If you would have told me that a visit to a surf therapy event in 2010 would have impacted the trajectory of my life—leading to two globally-distributed books—I wouldn't have believed you.

It was all based on the singular question: how is surfing therapeutic? The more I researched and the more I spoke with practitioners, the more it made sense: not only was surfing providing a natural euphoria thanks to dopamine flooding your limbic system. Surfing requires you to be in the moment—focusing on the present waves coming your direction—and not remembering traumas from the past, which provides a natural and blue-water escape. It's quite genius, really.

Even better, this in-the-moment, dopamine-rich experience is held in the ocean. Its color, texture and the fact that it envelops you from head to toe soothes, calms, relaxes...and washes away anything that you want to be rid of.

As you learn to surf with a surf therapy organization, you have a surf therapy practitioner and/or volunteer alongside you, helping you with instruction and catching waves, providing a desire to achieve the goal of standing and riding a wave. The practitioner and/or volunteer helps you because he or she has experienced many similar moments and similar traumas; because of this, there's an incredible trust and reliability factor. Besides receiving the euphoric benefits of surfing, you can open up and say how you truly feel because you will be heard and understood.

If that's not enough, you have a community of people cheering you on, providing words of affirmation and positive reinforcement as you ride waves according to your skill level. It's your own cheering arena, really—something that otherwise only professional athletes and movie stars experience in stadiums and on red carpets.

Just *one* of those instances by itself is therapeutic. Having all of them blended together? Well, that's surf therapy. A therapeutic scene, indeed!

Another set rose above the horizon that pulled me from my thoughts, and I found myself in the perfect spot for the first wave that dramatically increased in size as it rolled my direction. Paddling hard, I rose to my feet to see a glassy blue line elongating, an open canvas right before my eyes. I carved again and again until my legs burned and dismounted just as I was about to land on dry sand.

Paddling back out yet again, I thought about how surf therapy events have not only impacted my life. The same can be said for so many others who have attended surf therapy events all over the globe, whether they are practitioners, participants or volunteers. If you told each of them how much one surf therapy session would impact their lives, personally and professionally, they may not have believed you either.

That's what fascinated me most while writing this book. Nearly every practitioner who had become a member of the surf therapy sector, including its pioneers, experienced surfing as a form of therapy when they needed it the most. They were each curious how it had such a profound impact on themselves, and realized that if it could help them, it could help others going through the same experience.

And with that singular trait—a desire to give back— surf therapy has grown from a few volunteers and participants getting together onto the beach into a sector, with surf therapy events happening on any given day all over the world.

A set rose on the horizon, and I paddled to meet it. As I let the first wave go, I thought about how that trait has not only driven surf therapy to what it is today; it will continue to drive it in the years to come. The second wave looked like the best wave of the day, and I turned and paddled hard.

It was then, dropping in and seeing an endless ethereal blue line in front of me, that I realized above all, giving back—going to whatever lengths it takes to help others in need—will forever remain one of the most important traits for humans on earth.

ADVICE FOR SURF THERAPY PRACTITIONERS

In the process of writing this book, I spoke with more than two dozen surf therapy practitioners, many of whom are considered the pioneers of the sector itself. I asked them for advice for others in the sector. Here's what they had to say.

COLLECT DATA

Kris Primacio, CEO of ISTO:

> "First, surf therapy programs start with your heart—let that guide you in your acts of service. Second, practice collecting data. If research is outside your wheelhouse, collaborate with local universities to access expertise. You can connect with professors and students interested in collaborating on research projects by contacting researchers from different fields, such as psychology, occupational therapy, or sports psychology. Especially those students pursuing master's or Ph.D. degrees because they need research projects to fulfill their academic requirements. You can form a mutually beneficial partnership by allowing them to work on a project that aligns with your goals. They can provide

practical experience while you benefit from their expertise and assistance in collecting and analyzing data. Collaborating with universities can add credibility to your research endeavors. Most importantly, the partnership can lead to valuable insights and findings that contribute to the advancement of surf therapy."

GROW YOUR ORGANIZATION SLOW AND STEADY

Carly Rogers OTD, OTR/L:

"For existing therapists, grow it small and steady. Make sure you're making the impact you want before you grow and grow. How do you keep the integrity of the program and expand to get the monetary income to continue your program? Do you start to lose efficacy? Keep the integrity."

FOLLOW MEASUREMENT-BASED CARE

Kristen Walter, Clinical Research Psychologist and Division Head of the Clinical Research Program at the Naval Health Research Center in San Diego:

"We're in a mental health crisis right now. At the end of the day, if practitioners can provide surf therapy with care and compassion in whatever way they have the resources to do, that is above all my recommendation. If they can meet people where they're at and it's accessible, do what you can do with care and compassion. Second, if resources allow, try and have a regularly occurring program just be able to continue the benefit. Third, do some measurement based care. This means doing an ongoing assessment so you can use that to inform care delivery. It can be as simple as giving participants a piece of paper and asking

them to circle their mood before and after treatment, or you could do a ratings scale. Write a word of how you're feeling now, and how you're feeling after surfing. Have a child draw a picture before and after. You can make it as simple or complicated as you want. If someone isn't improving moods over the sessions, you want to know and talk to that person to see what's going on for them. Surf therapy is still evolving, and we're still learning what's important—what are the essential elements we need to be providing, and what things don't have an impact on outcome but might be a preference of the program. If you can get a sense of this, it allows the program to adapt and meet participants' needs. Doing measurement based care, whether it's simple or complicated, provides data so that you know how to alter your care."

BE BASED IN COMMUNITY

Natalie Small, Founder of Groundswell Community Project:

"Be based in community. As I've been training people to get their program started, ones not based off community are still successful, but there's more barriers because it's tough to get people on board. For those programs built off community, they blossom. When it comes to community, it's already happening. You're holding the space and people are already showing up. From my personal experience of how Groundswell has grown, it was all community. It started as an art therapy group with Generate Hope. I thought let's try surf therapy out and we did it because the women begged me to take them to the sea. It was not my idea—it was theirs! Our first surf therapy program was inspired by their deep desire to be in the sea for their healing. I was nervous, saw barriers, potential risk...but because of their perseverance, we overcame those barriers, took the risk,

and trusted. Now, because those eight women pursued their call to the sea for healing, over 4000 women and their communities around the world have also gotten the opportunity to take part in Groundswell surf therapy programs and reclaim their healing, power, and belonging in mother ocean as well. All of this exists because of those women, whom I am forever grateful for! As we grew, I needed fellow instructors, and girl friends started helping. Others came to experience it and became volunteers. More started coming and it kept growing. I was in a position of listening, saying yes and holding the space versus trying to make that space happen. For years we didn't have finances—but our community stepped up. While we were not abundant in finances, we were overflowing in abundance of support, volunteers, gear donations, and community! Even now we do not purchase new surfboards—all the gear we have has been donated by community members which also follows our ocean conservation value. This allows us to use our finances to create a valued and competitive pay for our all women staff and clinical facilitators so we can provide the best care possible for the communities we serve. That's the power of being based in community."

FOCUS ON ONE PARTICIPANT

Nick Hounsfeld, founder of The Wave:

"If you can use surfing to change just one person's life that is incredibly powerful...and if you then have the capacity to scale this up and have an impact on a far greater number of people, then that is really exciting. We have seen surf therapy in action at The Wave through our work with groups like The

Wave Project, but we also witness the positive power of being in waves every day on everyone who steps into our lake. It's what drives us. It's important to have a clear sense of purpose, and hopefully everybody in surf therapy is driven by a desire to make a positive impact on people's lives. It doesn't matter if it's for one person or hundreds of thousands of people—it's all about creating purposeful impact and democratizing blue health."

BE CHILD CENTRIC

Tom Losey, Founder of Liquid Therapy:

"Just be child-centric. That's what it comes back to every single time. Just let them lead. Just let them lead you. Don't make it about you helping them, just let them lead you. If you go in with the idea of helping, you have an idea of what you should be doing. And then you go a bit wrong from there because you've got the wrong mindset. If you get the volunteers together and say, 'Tell me your perfect wave,' one will say head high; another will say double overhead; another will say barreling...everyone has something different. If you rock up at Malibu and it's 2 feet and perfect, you'd think the kids will have the wave of their lives. But that's the wave of your life, not maybe theirs. It's very easy to get your influence on that session. Being child-centric, in that session, may be building sandcastles on the shore. The best sessions are the ones where afterwards, when the volunteer is like, 'Why is this kid here? He's normal.' He's normal because you just let him lead the session and there haven't been any barriers in his journey during that session. Disability isn't a disability; it's that the system isn't adapted to meet the needs."

SEEK MENTORSHIP FROM OTHER ORGANIZATIONS AND PROGRAMS

Eddie Donnellan, Founder of MeWater:

"My best advice is to reach out to a like-minded organization you're inspired by, talk to the leadership and pick their brains on how they started. Get advice. Get tough questions. Be persistent to speak to the founder or the leader. I'm giving this advice because I wish I had done it; I had no idea how to start an organization back then. Feel free to contact me. That's the mentorship aspect of MeWater that we promote."

HELP PARTICIPANTS FEEL COMFORTABLE AND SAFE

Dr. Jamie Marshall, Research Fellow at Edinburgh Napier University

"It's really about your population. Think about how you're going to make them comfortable, how to make them safe. Surfing is powerful, but if you can't help people feel comfortable or safe to talk or even try it, it loses that power. One of the examples from my own practice was a little girl who came to surf session. She got out of the car, and that was a huge achievement for her and we celebrated that. No expectation. If that's where you're going to get to today, well done, and we are here to support you when you are ready to try the next step. Really meeting people where they're at. Meet participants on the same level. Focus on getting rid of power structures—i.e., facilitator versus participant. In our research we developed the idea of participatory facilitation, where sharing vulnerability and building trust are key. Breaking down boundaries and stigma for clinician and patient, which is

something the medical world has wrestled with for a long time. When I was running volunteer training, I stressed it wasn't all about the surfing. You came to the beach to do surf therapy, and sometimes that means building sandcastles with someone to help them feel comfortable. It's just about meeting people where they are at and holding a truly safe space for participants."

BEFORE STARTING AN ORGANIZATION, CONSIDER A PARTNERSHIP WITH AN EXISTING ORGANIZATION

Joel Pilgrim, Founder of Waves of Wellness Foundation:

"If you want to start an organization, I would encourage you to think twice. So many organizations are doing wonderful things that we don't need more NGOs, we don't need more charities. We need to be smarter about how we work together. A lot of people are passionate about a cause and will want to be a founder of something. From my experience, things could have been different if we partnered with people. If you don't have a mental health professional background, training, or certification, find the people that do and partner with them."

DO SURF THERAPY BECAUSE YOU LOVE IT

Joe Taylor, Founder of the Wave Project:

"Do it because you love it. There has to be love in the work. You've got to really feel and empathize with the people you're supporting. That's where the fire comes from, the difference

you're making in their lives. That's what drove and continues to drive me. If you feel that's why you're doing it, everything else will fall into place."

HAVE FUN ON YOUR PARTICIPANT'S TERMS

Tim Conibear, Founder of Waves for Change:

"Listen to the people who are coming surfing with you and respond to their needs. From my own experience of going to see counselors, quite often, I felt that for the counselor to achieve their job they needed me to have a breakthrough. So, there's quite a push from the counselor to the person going through the experience. You can extend that metaphor to anything as a surf coach…you really want your student to stand up and feel better. For some kids going into the water for the first time up to their ankles is enough, and that's a huge win. That's therapeutic. They get confidence from it, and it builds a relationship with you. After eight times of doing that, they may have a conversation with you. Making sure the whole program is built around the wants of the kids or the adults or soldiers whoever is going to the beach. They are the experts and you're there to put them in the water any way they want to experience it. Try not to have any preconceived ideas of what surf therapy is, just take people to the beach, have fun. But have fun on their terms."

WORK WITH EXPERTS IN THE FIELD

Joel Pilgrim, Founder of Waves of Wellness Foundation:

"Bring in experts who have that track record of supporting the mental health journey. We have a duty of care. We're not

just going for a surf here. We're dealing with people who are incredibly vulnerable. We need to make sure we're not doing surf therapy in a detrimental way, putting people at risk of exacerbating their mental health condition."

REALIZE THAT WE ARE PART OF THE OCEAN

Easkey Britton, author of *Saltwater in the Blood: Surfing, Natural Cycles and the Sea's Power to Heal*

"With my research background in blue health, my role very much has been about facilitating those who want to deliver surf therapy programs. I'm increasingly seeing pressure for more funding, and the challenges therein... The pressure to capture impact and measure and evaluate the human health outcomes. My hope is that this doesn't come at the cost of commodifying the ocean, or over medicalizing it. Instead of asking what the ocean can do for us or how can the ocean heal us, what if we recognized that we are part of the ocean? That as the ocean works its restorative powers on us, we must also work to restore the ocean's health. If we don't also foster this culture of care and reciprocity within surf therapy we run the risk of perpetuating society and culture of dominance over nature, that is ultimately leading to the destruction of our own health and wellbeing. The ocean is a key actor and player in this healing process, and I think it's important to see that acknowledged and reflected more strongly in the research and programmatic language, aims and outcomes."

HAVE A TRAINED WATER TEAM

Operation Surf:

> *"Your water team is paramount to your success. Having quality surf structures, water safety, having your water team knowing what they're doing can make or break a program. You could potentially send someone into more trauma by not having someone who knows what they're doing. Invest in that with someone who is just starting out."*

FOLLOW THESE THREE TIERS

Carly Rogers OTD, OTR/L:

> *"If you're developing a program, I feel there needs to be three tiers. You need a supportive body with access to equipment and surf instructors such as a surf school, a therapeutic agent, whoever is going to lead it, and connecting with a university for program evaluation is helpful."*

SURF THERAPY RESOURCE GUIDE

I f these surf therapy stories have inspired you to take the next step, whether that's volunteering, becoming a participant, or getting involved in the surf therapy sector, the next question is where to start.

Because of such rapid growth of the sector at large, there are organizations worldwide that are likely near you. Here's how to get in contact with them.

Ability Surf: Based in New South Wales, Ability Surf combines the medicine of the ocean and surfing with person-person connection to enable all people equal opportunity to access the ocean in a supportive and caring environment. Their mission is to create a more inclusive community, supporting people with a disability and their support networks to feel acknowledged, seen and supported. Visit abilitysurf. com.au/ for more information.

Amp Surf: The Association of Amputee Surfers promotes, inspires, educates, and rehabilitates all people with disabilities, including veterans, and first Responders through Adaptive Surf Therapy and other outdoor activities. The organization has four chapters throughout the

United States: California, New England, New York, and the Pacific Northwest. Visit AmpSurf.org for more information.

A Walk on Water: Based in Southern California, AWOW Surf Therapy creates positive, uplifting, and empowering surf therapy experiences. In addition to surf therapy, their events offer yoga, massage therapy, art therapy, music therapy, food and drink, and many different variations of sport and play on the beach. Visit AWalkonWater.org for more information.

Best Day Foundation: Based in Virginia, The Best Day Foundation enables children and young adults with special needs to build confidence and self-esteem through adventure activities which stretch their limits, expand their true potential, reinforce their achievement, and connect them with diverse populations in their community. Learn more at bestdayfoundation.org.

City Surf Project: The City Surf Project ensures youth in the San Francisco Bay Area have equitable access to the ocean through surf instruction. They use surfing as a vehicle to improve the health and well-being of our youth. Learn more at CitySurfProject.com.

Disfrutar El Mar: Headquartered in Spain, Disfrutar El Mar uses surfing as a tool for the integral development and autonomy of children in a playful way, promoting sensory-motor, psychomotor, social, and emotional capacities. Visit Disfrutarelmar.org for more information.

Waves of Wellness Foundation: Waves of Wellness (WOW) Foundation is a mental health surf therapy charity serving Australia, committed to changing lives by delivering for-purpose, innovative support programs for people experiencing mental health challenges. Visit FoundationWow.org for more information.

Gnome Surf: Located in Rhode Island, Gnome Surf focuses on creating a culture shift towards happiness, kindness, love, and acceptance for all kids of all abilities regardless of socio economic status through life changing surf therapy, art therapy, yoga and eco-therapy experiences. Visit Gnomesurf.com for more information.

Groundswell Community Project: A research-based trauma informed surf therapy non-profit organization, the Groundswell Community Project provides a safe and resilient community for all identifying as women on their healing journey. With our home roots in San Diego, California, and community partnerships that extend across the globe, the non-profit organization strives to break down barriers and build up communities that celebrate mental health and ocean health. Visit GroundswellCommunity.org for more information.

Jimmy Miller Memorial Foundation: Located in Los Angeles, the Jimmy Miller Memorial Foundation (JMMF) is an adaptive surfing program to assist individuals coping with mental and physical illness in accessing the ocean environment. The purpose of the program is to increase perceived self-efficacy in participants, through engagement in physical activity in the ocean environment, specifically, the activity of surfing. Visit jimmymillerfoundation.org for more information.

International Surf Therapy Organization: The global community of surf therapy practitioners and researchers, ISTO harnesses the power of collaboration and the ocean to advance the use of surf therapy as a mental and physical health intervention. The International Surf Therapy Organization facilitates high impact research on the effectiveness of surf therapy. Visit intlsurftherapy.org for more information.

Ocean Mind: A therapeutic surfing charity that enriches people's mental health, relationships and potential through surfing, Ocean Mind is committed to developing evidence-based programs that create life-changing experiences for people experiencing mental health challenges, social isolation and disabilities. Ocean Mind is located in Australia. Visit Oceanmind.org.au for more information.

One More Wave: Based in San Diego, One More Wave's mission is to provide wounded and disabled veterans with customized surfing equipment and a community to surf with. By equipping veterans and connecting them to a global network of surfing volunteers, One More Wave empowers veterans to heal through surf therapy from coast to coast. Visit Onemorewave.com for more information.

Liquid Therapy: Based in Ireland, Liquid Therapy is a multi-award winning charity which provides inclusive and adaptive surf therapy programs which are beneficial to our physical and mental health. Their mission is that the mental health and wellbeing benefits of the Ocean and surfing are available to all. Visit LiquidTherapy.ie for more information.

Live for More: Located in New Zealand, Live For More's purpose is to empower young people to find freedom from their troubled pasts and be inspired to live positive and fulfilling lives. Through their surf therapy programs, they transform troubled lives one wave at a time. Visit LiveForMore.org.nz for more information.

MeWater: MeWater connects at-risk youth to the healing power of the ocean through surf therapy by surfers and mental health professionals in the San Francisco Bay Area. They provide day and overnight surf camps to youth, families, and groups, with a mental health approach to mindfulness, empowerment, and exposure to the ocean and the great outdoors. Visit MeWaterFoundation.org for more information.

Operation Surf: Based in California, Operation Surf's mission is to channel the healing powers of the ocean to restore hope, renew purpose, and revitalize community. Operation Surf's curriculum-based programs aim to inspire injured military and veterans to seek wellness in all aspects of their lives while providing the necessary resources, tools, and peer-to-peer support to continue this mindset indefinitely. Visit operationsurf.org for more information.

Roxy Davis Foundation: The Roxy Davis Foundation aims to affect meaningful evidence-based change in people's lives by improving their mental and physical well-being through ocean based therapy programs. The Foundation is based in South Africa. For more information, visit RoxyDavisfoundation.org.

Surfers for Autism: Surfers for Autism unlocks the potential of children and adults with autism, building awareness and uniting communities through volunteerism in Florida. Visit SurfersforAutism.org for more information.

Surfers Healing: The original surf camp for children with autism, Surfer's Healing is based in California but hosts events around the globe. It serves to enrich the lives of people living with autism by exposing them to the unique experience of surfing. Visit SurfersHealing.org for more information.

Surfing the Spectrum: A Surf Therapy initiative in Australia, Surfing the Spectrum works to positively impact the lives of families, and their children with Autism. Visit SurfingtheSpectrum.org for more information.

Surf and Turf Foundation: The Surf and Turf Therapy Foundation provides therapy services targeting traditional, functional goals using non-traditional approaches, including surfing, horseback riding and community-based activities in California. Visit Surfandturftherapy.org for more information.

Surf Addict Portugal: One of the first adapted surfing associations in Europe, Portuguese Association of Adapted Surfing intends to make surfing available to people with any type of limitation, be it motor, visual or cognitive. Visit Surfadaptado.pt for more information.

Surf and Durf: Located in the Netherlands, Surf and Durf uses wave surfing as a medium in the implementation of psychological treatment programs. Visit Stichtingsurfendurf.nl for more information.

Surfivor: Located in the Netherlands, Surfivor uses surf therapy to help those who struggle with PTSD get out of the negative spiral, to get a sense of life again, to take on challenges and to go for it. For more information, visit surfivor.nl.

SurfTherapie: SurfTherapie uses surf therapy to help those in rehabilitation after a neurological disorder, such as brain injury. Visit Surftherapie.nl for more information.

Surfwell: Surfwell delivers surf therapy for blue light services across England with a highly trained team who hold nationally recognised water safety and mental health qualifications. Visit Surfwell.co.uk for more information.

Urban Surf 4 Kids: Based in California, Urban Surf 4 Kids provide opportunities for healing and empowerment through surf therapy, mentorship, and life skills achievement programs for youth in foster and at-risk communities. Learn more at Urbansurf4kids.org.

Warrior Surf Foundation: The Warrior Surf Foundation exists to provide free surf therapy, wellness coaching, yoga, and community to Veterans struggling with PTSD, anxiety, depression, transition issues, and other mental health issues. Located in South Carolina, the Foundation believes that all Veterans deserve the right to live lives to their fullest potential. Visit WarriorSurf.org for more information.

The Wave Project: The world's "first 'surf therapy' course funded by a government health service," The Wave Project harnesses the power of the ocean to improve the mental health of children and young people in the UK. Their 6,000 volunteer surf mentors deliver life-changing surf therapy every day. Visit the WaveProject.co.uk for more information.

Waves for Change: Waves for Change provides child-friendly mental health services to children and young people in under-resourced communities in South Africa and beyond. Visit Waves-for-Change.org.

Waves 4 Women: Waves 4 Women empowers women to build emotional and physical wellness as well as safe supportive communities through a combination of surf instruction, women's wellness groups, and community building. Visit Waves4women.org for more information.

Wirmachenwelle: Wirmachenwelle brings young people from Germany's cities onto the surfboard and into nature to increase their well-being, make them strong and have a lasting influence on the development of their personal resources and social skills. For more information, visit wirmachenwelle.org.

BIBLIOGRAPHY

eee

CHAPTER 1

1.   McPhillips, Deidre. "90 percent of US Adults Say the United States Is Experiencing a Mental Health Crisis, CNN/KFF Poll Finds." CNN, 5 Oct. 2022, www.cnn.com/2022/10/05/health/cnn-kff-mental-health-poll-wellness/index.html.

2.   Vogt, Dawne. "Research on Women, Trauma and PTSD." National Center for PTSD, U.S. Department of Veterans Affairs, 2023, www.ptsd.va.gov/professional/treat/specific/ptsd_research_women.asp.

3.   Centers for Disease Control and Prevention. "Data & Statistics on Autism Spectrum Disorder." CDC, 2023, www.cdc.gov/ncbddd/autism/data.html.

4.   World Health Organization. "World Report on Disability." World Health Organization, 2011, www.who.int/disabilities/world_report/2011/en/.

5.   UNHCR - United Nations High Commissioner for Refugees. "Figures at a Glance." UNHCR, https://www.unhcr.org/about-unhcr/who-we-are/figures-glance.

6.   "International Surf Therapy Organization." International Surf Therapy Organization, https://intlsurftherapy.org/.

7.   Lambert, Cash. "Surfing for a Cure." The Beacon: The Student Newspaper of Palm Beach Atlantic University, 8 Nov. 2010, pp. 1 & 8.

8.   Lambert, Cash. "Surfing for a Cure." The Beacon: The Student Newspaper of Palm Beach Atlantic University, 8 Nov. 2010, pp. 1 & 8.

9. Lambert, Cash. "International Surf Therapy Symposium Breaks Ground in LA." International Surf Therapy Symposium Breaks Ground in LA, Surfline, Oct. 2019, https://www.surfline.com/surf-news/international-surf-therapy-symposium-breaks-ground-la/69504.

10. Lambert, Cash. "International Surf Therapy Symposium Breaks Ground in LA." International Surf Therapy Symposium Breaks Ground in LA, Surfline, Oct. 2019, https://www.surfline.com/surf-news/international-surf-therapy-symposium-breaks-ground-la/69504.

11. Smith, J. T. (2016). Illustrated Atlas of Surfing History. Island Heritage Publishing. pp. 45.

12. Ho'oulumahiehie, & Nogelmeier, M. P. (2021). The Epic Tale of Hi'ikaikapoliopele (M. P. Nogelmeier, Trans.). Honolulu, HI: University of Hawai'i Press. pp. 218-222.

13. "Blind Catch a Wave at Surfing School." Los Angeles Times, 24 July 1988, www.latimes.com/archives/la-xpm-1988-07-24-mn-10469-story.html.

14. "Blind Youngsters Learn How to Conquer the Waves ." San Francisco Chronicle, 1986.

15. "Blind Catch a Wave at Surfing School." Los Angeles Times, 24 July 1988, www.latimes.com/archives/la-xpm-1988-07-24-mn-10469-story.html.

16. " Sea Me, Feel Me: Blind Kids Slide Malibu." Surfer Magazine, circa 1989. pp 33.

17. Silverberg, Ted. "Give a Little Bit Back ."

18. Primacio, Kris. "Surfer Kris Primacio Turns a Personal Refuge into a Way to Heal Others in Need." Golden State, Golden State, 13 Mar. 2022, goldenstate.is/surfer-kris-primacio-turns-a-personal-refuge-into-a-way-to-heal-others-in-need/.

19. Primacio, Kris. "Surfer Kris Primacio Turns a Personal Refuge into a Way to Heal Others in Need." Golden State, Golden State, 13 Mar. 2022, goldenstate.is/surfer-kris-primacio-turns-a-personal-refuge-into-a-way-to-heal-others-in-need/.

20. Marshall, J. A Global Exploration of Programme Theory within Surf Therapy. (Thesis). Edinburgh Napier University. Retrieved from http://researchrepository.napier.ac.uk/Output/2879652

21. Sarkisian, Gregor V. "Dr. Sarkisian Coedits a Special Issue of 'Global Journal of Community Psychology Practice'." Common Thread, Antioch University, 14 Jan. 2023, commonthread.antioch.edu/dr-sarkisian-coedits-a-special-issue-of-global-journal-of-community-psychology-practice/.

22. Benninger, Elizabeth, Chloe Curtis, Gregor V. Sarkisian, Carly M. Rogers, Kailey Bender, and Megan Comer. "Surf Therapy: A Scoping Review of the Qualitative and Quantitative Research Evidence." Global Journal of Community Psychology Practice 11, no. 2 (2020): 206-223. https://www.gjcpp.org/en/article.php?issue=36&article=206.

23. Benninger, Elizabeth, Chloe Curtis, Gregor V. Sarkisian, Carly M. Rogers, Kailey Bender, and Megan Comer. "Surf Therapy: A Scoping Review of the Qualitative and Quantitative Research Evidence." Global Journal of Community Psychology Practice 11, no. 2 (2020): 206-223. https://www.gjcpp.org/en/article.php?issue=36&article=206.

24. Benninger, Elizabeth, Chloe Curtis, Gregor V. Sarkisian, Carly M. Rogers, Kailey Bender, and Megan Comer. "Surf Therapy: A Scoping Review of the Qualitative and Quantitative Research Evidence." Global Journal of Community Psychology Practice 11, no. 2 (2020): 206-223. https://www.gjcpp.org/en/article.php?issue=36&article=206.

25. Benninger, Elizabeth, Chloe Curtis, Gregor V. Sarkisian, Carly M. Rogers, Kailey Bender, and Megan Comer. "Surf Therapy: A Scoping Review of the Qualitative and Quantitative Research Evidence." Global Journal of Community Psychology Practice 11, no. 2 (2020): 206-223. https://www.gjcpp.org/en/article.php?issue=36&article=206.

26. Benninger, Elizabeth, Chloe Curtis, Gregor V. Sarkisian, Carly M. Rogers, Kailey Bender, and Megan Comer. "Surf Therapy: A Scoping Review of the Qualitative and Quantitative Research Evidence." Global Journal of Community Psychology Practice 11, no. 2 (2020): 206-223. https://www.gjcpp.org/en/article.php?issue=36&article=206.

27. Marshall, J. A Global Exploration of Programme Theory within Surf Therapy. (Thesis). Edinburgh Napier University. Retrieved from http://researchrepository.napier.ac.uk/Output/2879652

28. Marshall, J. A Global Exploration of Programme Theory within Surf Therapy. (Thesis). Edinburgh Napier University. Retrieved from http://researchrepository.napier.ac.uk/Output/2879652

CHAPTER 2

29. "Surfing—Infinite Possibilities to Heal | Carly Rogers | TEDxUCLA." YouTube, YouTube, 3 July 2014, https://www.youtube.com/watch?v=Wfb8tHn8Xv4.

30. "Surfing—Infinite Possibilities to Heal | Carly Rogers | TEDxUCLA." YouTube, YouTube, 3 July 2014, https://www.youtube.com/watch?v=Wfb8tHn8Xv4.

31. "Jimmy's Legacy." Jimmy Miller Foundation, 11 Mar. 2023, jimmymillerfoundation. org/jimmys-legacy/.

32. "Jimmy's Legacy." Jimmy Miller Foundation, 11 Mar. 2023, jimmymillerfoundation. org/jimmys-legacy/.

33. "Jimmy's Legacy." Jimmy Miller Foundation, 11 Mar. 2023, jimmymillerfoundation. org/jimmys-legacy/.

34. "Surfing—Infinite Possibilities to Heal | Carly Rogers | TEDxUCLA." YouTube, YouTube, 3 July 2014, https://www.youtube.com/watch?v=Wfb8tHn8Xv4.

35. Skenazy, Matt, et al. "Can Surfing Reprogram the Veteran's Brain?" Outside Online, 1 Nov. 2021, www.outsideonline.com/outdoor-adventure/water-activities/ trim-toward-light-ptsd-surf-therapy/.

36. "Surfing—Infinite Possibilities to Heal | Carly Rogers | TEDxUCLA." YouTube, YouTube, 3 July 2014, https://www.youtube.com/watch?v=Wfb8tHn8Xv4.

37. "Surfing—Infinite Possibilities to Heal | Carly Rogers | TEDxUCLA." YouTube, YouTube, 3 July 2014, https://www.youtube.com/watch?v=Wfb8tHn8Xv4.

38. "Surfing—Infinite Possibilities to Heal | Carly Rogers | TEDxUCLA." YouTube, YouTube, 3 July 2014, https://www.youtube.com/watch?v=Wfb8tHn8Xv4.

39. "Jimmy Miller Memorial Foundation Guidestar Pro Report." Jimmy Miller Memorial Foundation, 14 Jan. 2023, jimmymillerfoundation.org/wp-content/ uploads/2023/03/Candid-GuideStar-JMMF-Report-2022.pdf.

40. "Surfing—Infinite Possibilities to Heal | Carly Rogers | TEDxUCLA." YouTube, YouTube, 3 July 2014, https://www.youtube.com/watch?v=Wfb8tHn8Xv4.

41. "Surfing—Infinite Possibilities to Heal | Carly Rogers | TEDxUCLA." YouTube, YouTube, 3 July 2014, https://www.youtube.com/watch?v=Wfb8tHn8Xv4.

42. Rogers, Carly M, et al. "High-Intensity Sports for Posttraumatic Stress Disorder and Depression: Feasibility Study of Ocean Therapy with Veterans of Operation Enduring Freedom and Operation Iraqi Freedom." The American Journal of Occupational Therapy : Official Publication of the American Occupational Therapy Association, 2014, pubmed.ncbi.nlm.nih.gov/25005502/.

43. Fleischmann, David, et al. Surf Medicine: Surfing as a Means of Therapy for Combat-Related Polytrauma, 2011, www.researchgate.net/publication/232113675_ Surf_Medicine_Surfing_as_a_Means_of_Therapy_for_Combat-Related_Polytrauma.

44. Fleischmann, David, et al. Surf Medicine: Surfing as a Means of Therapy for Combat-Related Polytrauma, 2011, www.researchgate.net/publication/232113675_Surf_Medicine_Surfing_as_a_Means_of_Therapy_for_Combat-Related_Polytrauma.

45. Blakeley, Katherine, and Don J. Jansen. "Post-Traumatic Stress Disorder and Other Mental Health Problems in the Military: Oversight Issues for Congress." CRS Report R43088, Congressional Research Service, 8 Aug. 2013, fas.org/sgp/crs/natsec/R43088.pdf.

46. Walter, Kristen H, et al. "Breaking the Surface: Psychological Outcomes among U.S. Active Duty Service Members Following a Surf Therapy Program." Psychology of Sport and Exercise, 18 June 2019, www.sciencedirect.com/science/article/abs/pii/S1469029219301372.

47. Glassman, Lisa H, et al. "Gender Differences in Psychological Outcomes Following Surf Therapy Sessions among U.S. Service Members." International Journal of Environmental Research and Public Health, 2021, pubmed.ncbi.nlm.nih.gov/33925447/.

48. Walter, Kristen H., Nicholas P. Otis, Travis N. Ray, Lisa H. Glassman, Jessica L. Beltran, et al. "A Randomized Controlled Trial of Surf and Hike Therapy for U.S. Active Duty Service Members with Major Depressive Disorder - BMC Psychiatry." BMC Psychiatry, 17 Feb. 2023, bmcpsychiatry.biomedcentral.com/articles/10.1186/s12888-022-04452-7

49. Manzi, Andrew. "CNN Hero Andrew Manzi: Warrior Surf." CNN, 31 Aug. 2017, www.cnn.com/2017/08/31/health/cnn-hero-andrew-manzi-warrior-surf/index.html.

50. Manzi, Andrew. "CNN Heroes: Top 10 - Andrew Manzi." CNN, 7 Nov. 2017, www.cnn.com/videos/tv/2017/11/07/cnn-heroes-top-10-manzi-orig-mc.cnn.

51. "Warrior Surf Foundation - CNN Heroes Nomination Andy Manzi." YouTube, YouTube, 8 Dec. 2017, https://www.youtube.com/watch?v=9fD0ciljvjM.

52. "About." Warrior Surf, www.warriorsurf.org/about.

53. "About." Warrior Surf, www.warriorsurf.org/about.

54. Young, Harmony of Illusions, 7

55. Alan Zerembo, "As Disability Awards Grow, So Do Concerns with Veracity of PTSD Claims," Los Angeles Times, August 3, 2014.

56. Richard J. McNally and B. Christopher Frueh, "Why Are Iraq and Afghanistan War Veterans Seeking PTSD Disability Compensation at Unprecedented Rates?," Journal of Anxiety Disorders 27 (2013: 520-526, 520

57. "Va.Gov: Veterans Affairs." Moral Injury, 20 Apr. 2020, www.ptsd.va.gov/professional/treat/cooccurring/moral_injury.asp.

58. "Va.Gov: Veterans Affairs." Moral Injury, 20 Apr. 2020, www.ptsd.va.gov/professional/treat/cooccurring/moral_injury.asp.

59. Grossman, Dave. On Killing: The Psychological Cost of Learning to Kill in War and Society. Little, Brown and Company, 1995, pp. xxxv.

60. Grossman, Dave. On Killing: The Psychological Cost of Learning to Kill in War and Society. Little, Brown and Company, 1995, pp. 74.

61. "Overview of VA Research on Posttraumatic Stress Disorder (PTSD)." Posttraumatic Stress Disorder (PTSD), www.research.va.gov/topics/ptsd.cfm.

62. "WARRIOR SURF FOUNDATION." Warrior Surf, www.warriorsurf.org/.

63. "WARRIOR SURF FOUNDATION." Warrior Surf, www.warriorsurf.org/.

64. "If They Are Dreaming of the Waves Tomorrow, They Won't Take Their Life Today. Operation Surf." Operation Surf, 21 Feb. 2023, operationsurf.org/.

65. "Hidden Pearls Podcast - Operation Surf - Van Curaza, Amanda Curaza & Justin Martinez." YouTube, YouTube, 30 Aug. 2022, https://www.youtube.com/watch?v=WNCfpp6NKiI.

66. Grossman, Dave. On Killing: The Psychological Cost of Learning to Kill in War and Society. Little, Brown and Company, 1995, pp. 149.

67. Grossman, Dave. On Killing: The Psychological Cost of Learning to Kill in War and Society. Little, Brown and Company, 1995, pp. 89.

68. "Resurface." Netflix, 2017, https://www.netflix.com/title/80184055.

69. "Resurface." Netflix, 2017, https://www.netflix.com/title/80184055.

70. "If They Are Dreaming of the Waves Tomorrow, They Won't Take Their Life Today. Operation Surf." Operation Surf, 21 Feb. 2023, operationsurf.org/.

71. Crawford, Russell Todd. The Impact of Ocean Therapy with Posttraumatic Stress Disorder, 2023. Print. pp 29.

72. Crawford, Russell Todd. The Impact of Ocean Therapy with Posttraumatic Stress Disorder, 2023. Print. pp 35.

73. Crawford, Russell Todd. The Impact of Ocean Therapy with Posttraumatic Stress Disorder, 2023. Print. pp 35.

74. Crawford, Russell Todd. The Impact of Ocean Therapy with Posttraumatic Stress Disorder, 2023. Print. pp 31

75. Ossie, J. E. (2023). Utilizing New Technologies to Measure Therapy Effectiveness for Mental and Physical Health (Doctoral dissertation, University of San Diego).

76. Ossie, J. E. (2023). Utilizing New Technologies to Measure Therapy Effectiveness for Mental and Physical Health (Doctoral dissertation, University of San Diego).

77. Ossie, J. E. (2023). Utilizing New Technologies to Measure Therapy Effectiveness for Mental and Physical Health (Doctoral dissertation, University of San Diego).

CHAPTER 3

78. TEDxTalks. "Surf Therapy - A Wave of Change | Tim Conibear | Ted X Cape Town." YouTube, YouTube, 23 Jan. 2018, https://www.youtube.com/watch?v=tkqJmH0oEP0.

79. TEDxTalks. "Surf Therapy - A Wave of Change | Tim Conibear | Ted X Cape Town." YouTube, YouTube, 23 Jan. 2018, https://www.youtube.com/watch?v=tkqJmH0oEP0.

80. TEDxTalks. "Surf Therapy - A Wave of Change | Tim Conibear | Ted X Cape Town." YouTube, YouTube, 23 Jan. 2018, https://www.youtube.com/watch?v=tkqJmH0oEP0.

81. TEDxTalks. "Surf Therapy - A Wave of Change | Tim Conibear | Ted X Cape Town." YouTube, YouTube, 23 Jan. 2018, https://www.youtube.com/watch?v=tkqJmH0oEP0.

82. "Waves for Change - 10 Years of SURF THERAPY." YouTube, YouTube, 26 Oct. 2022, https://www.youtube.com/watch?v=rMa1ENla2wE&t=128s.

83. Authors, All, and Elizabeth Benninger MA & Shazly Savahl PhD. "The Use of Visual Methods to Explore How Children Construct and Assign Meaning to the 'Self' within Two Urban Communities in the Western Cape, South Africa." Taylor & Francis, https://www.tandfonline.com/doi/full/10.3402/qhw.v11.31251.

84. Authors, All, and Elizabeth Benninger MA & Shazly Savahl PhD. "The Use of Visual Methods to Explore How Children Construct and Assign Meaning to the 'Self' within Two Urban Communities in the Western Cape, South Africa." Taylor & Francis, https://www.tandfonline.com/doi/full/10.3402/qhw.v11.31251.

85. Authors, All, and Elizabeth Benninger MA & Shazly Savahl PhD. "The Use of Visual Methods to Explore How Children Construct and Assign Meaning to the 'Self' within Two Urban Communities in the Western Cape, South Africa." Taylor & Francis, https://www.tandfonline.com/doi/full/10.3402/qhw.v11.31251.

86. Waves for Change. "Closing the Mental Health Treatment Gap in South Africa: A Waves for Change Learning Brief." Waves for Change, 2022.

87. "How Toxic Stress Affects Children Living in Township Communities." Waves for Change, 22 Oct. 2021, waves-for-change.org/how-toxic-stress-affects-children-living-in-township-communities/.

88. Waves for Change. "Annual Report 2021". Waves for Change, 2021.

89. Waves for Change. "Annual Report 2021". Waves for Change, 2021.

90. Waves for Change. "Annual Report 2021". Waves for Change, 2021.

91. Waves for Change. "Closing the Mental Health Treatment Gap in South Africa: A Waves for Change Learning Brief." Waves for Change, 2022.

92. Waves for Change. "Closing the Mental Health Treatment Gap in South Africa: A Waves for Change Learning Brief." Waves for Change, 2022.

93. Waves for Change. "Waves for Change Learning Brief: HRV."

94. Waves for Change. "Waves for Change Learning Brief: HRV."

95. Waves for Change. "Waves for Change Learning Brief: HRV."

96. Waves for Change. "Waves for Change Learning Brief: HRV."

97. "Waves for Change - 10 Years of SURF THERAPY." YouTube, YouTube, 26 Oct. 2022, https://www.youtube.com/watch?v=rMa1ENla2wE&t=128s.

98. Waves for Change. "Waves for Change Annual Report: 2021."

99. "The Wave Alliance: What We Do." Waves for Change, 11 July 2022, waves-for-change.org/what-we-do/the-wave-alliance/.

100. Marshall, Jamie, et al. "'I Feel Happy When I Surf Because It Takes Stress from My Mind': An Initial Exploration of Program Theory within Waves for Change Surf Therapy in Post-Conflict Liberia." Journal of Sport for Development, vol. 9, no. 1, 1 Nov. 2020, https://doi.org/https://jsfd.org/2020/11/01/i-feel-happy-when-i-surf-because-it-takes-stress-from-my-mind-an-initial-exploration-of-program-theory-within-waves-for-change-surf-therapy-in-post-conflict-liberia/.

101. Marshall , Jamie, et al. "A Mixed Methods Exploration of Surf Therapy Piloted for Youth Well-Being in Post-Conflict Sierra Leone." International Journal of Environmental Research and Public Health, 10 June 2021, https://www.mdpi.com/1660-4601/18/12/6267.

102. Halloran, Cathy. "120 Chernobyl Children Arrive for Respite Break." RTE.Ie, 25 June 2019, www.rte.ie/news/munster/2019/0625/1057411-chernobyl-children/.

103.   International Atomic Energy Agency, World Health Organization, and European Commission. Ten Years After Chernobyl: What Do We Really Know? Proceedings of the IAEA/WHO/EC International Conference, Vienna, April 1996. International Atomic Energy Agency, 1996.

104.   "Chernobyl Will Be Unhabitable for at Least 3,000 Years, Say Nuclear Experts." The Christian Science Monitor, 24 Apr. 2016, www.csmonitor.com/World/Global-News/2016/0424/Chernobyl-will-be-unhabitable-for-at-least-3-000-years-say-nuclear-experts.

105.   "Chernobyl." Chernobyl Childrens Project UK, www.chernobyl-children.org.uk/the-effects-on-the-environment.

106.   Halloran, Cathy. "120 Chernobyl Children Arrive for Respite Break." RTE.Ie, 25 June 2019, www.rte.ie/news/munster/2019/0625/1057411-chernobyl-children/.

107.   Britton, Easkey. Saltwater in the Blood: Surfing, Natural Cycles and the Sea's Power to Heal, Watkins, London, 2021. pp 98.

108.   Halloran, Cathy. "120 Chernobyl Children Arrive for Respite Break." RTE.Ie, 25 June 2019, www.rte.ie/news/munster/2019/0625/1057411-chernobyl-children/.

109.   "Recuperative Holidays." Chernobyl Children's Project UK, www.chernobyl-children.org.uk/recuperative-holidays.

110.   Dickerson, Bryan. "2022 Update: The Big List of Prices and Times for All the World's Wave Pools." Wave Pool Magazine - For Your Curiosity and Stoke, 24 Apr. 2023, wavepoolmag.com/the-big-list-prices-times-notes-for-all-the-worlds-wave-pools/.

111.   "Who Is Low-Income and Very Low Income in the Bay Area?: Bay Area Equity Atlas." Who Is Low-Income and Very Low Income in the Bay Area? | Bay Area Equity Atlas, 21 Sept. 2020, bayareaequityatlas.org/node/60841.

112.   Fish People. Directed by Keith Malloy, Patagonia Films, 2020. YouTube, www.youtube.com/watch?v=lW1OHf_aBX0.

113.   Fish People. Directed by Keith Malloy, Patagonia Films, 2020. YouTube, www.youtube.com/watch?v=lW1OHf_aBX0.

114.   Mewater Brings Surfing and Mentorship to San Francisco's ... - Surfline, www.surfline.com/surf-news/mewater-brings-surfing-mentorship-san-franciscos-hunters-point/151930.

115.   Mewater Brings Surfing and Mentorship to San Francisco's ... - Surfline, www.surfline.com/surf-news/mewater-brings-surfing-mentorship-san-franciscos-hunters-point/151930.

116. "A Pandemic Can't Stop Mewater." Patagonia Stories, 18 Nov. 2021, www. patagonia.com/stories/a-pandemic-cant-stop-mewater/story-96608.html.

117. Fish People. Directed by Keith Malloy, Patagonia Films, 2020. YouTube, www. youtube.com/watch?v=lW1OHf_aBX0.

118. Fish People. Directed by Keith Malloy, Patagonia Films, 2020. YouTube, www. youtube.com/watch?v=lW1OHf_aBX0.

CHAPTER 4

119. Groundswell Community Project. "Groundswell Community Project." www. groundswellcommunity.org/.

120. "Women Who Experience Trauma Are Twice as Likely as Men to Develop PTSD. Here's Why." American Psychological Association, www.apa.org/topics/ women-girls/women-trauma.

121. Groundswell Community Project. "Groundswell Community Project." www. groundswellcommunity.org/.

122. "Trainings." Groundswell Community Project, www.groundswellcommunity.org/ groundswell-trainings.

123. "Trainings." Groundswell Community Project, www.groundswellcommunity.org/ groundswell-trainings.

124. Wave Wahines. Wave Wahines, wavewahines.co.uk/.

125. "Bio." Easkey Britton, 30 Mar. 2023, easkeybritton.com/bio/.

126. Britton, Easkey. Saltwater in the Blood: Surfing, Natural Cycles and the Sea's Power to Heal. Watkins, 2021. Pp 96.

127. Britton, Easkey. Saltwater in the Blood: Surfing, Natural Cycles and the Sea's Power to Heal. Watkins, 2021. Pp 94.

128. "History." Finisterre, finisterre.com/en-us/pages/history.

129. "Into the Sea: The Seasuit Project." Finisterre, finisterre.com/en-us/blogs/ broadcast/into-the-sea-the-finisterre-seasuit-project.

130. "Seasuit Products." Finisterre, finisterre.com/collections/seasuit.

131. "Swim Hijab Head Covering (Geometric Print)." Finisterre, finisterre.com/ products/into-the-sea-hijab-recycled-geometric-print.

132. Britton, Easkey. Saltwater in the Blood: Surfing, Natural Cycles and the Sea's Power to Heal. Watkins, 2021. Pp 205.

133. Britton, Easkey. Saltwater in the Blood: Surfing, Natural Cycles and the Sea's Power to Heal. Watkins, 2021. Pp 202.

134. Britton, Easkey. Saltwater in the Blood: Surfing, Natural Cycles and the Sea's Power to Heal. Watkins, 2021. Pp 202.

CHAPTER 5

135. "The Drop: How The Most Addictive Sport Can Help Us Understand Addiction and Recovery." Harper Wave, 2021, p. 106.

136. Waves of Freedom." Vimeo, uploaded by Dash Media, 19 Dec. 2019, vimeo.com/ondemand/wavesoffreedom/380658552.

137. Waves of Freedom." Vimeo, uploaded by Dash Media, 19 Dec. 2019, vimeo.com/ondemand/wavesoffreedom/380658552.

138. Waves of Freedom." Vimeo, uploaded by Dash Media, 19 Dec. 2019, vimeo.com/ondemand/wavesoffreedom/380658552.

139. Boomen, Marcus. "Where New Zealand Stands Internationally: A Comparison of Offence Profiles and Recidivism Rates." Practice: The New Zealand Corrections Journal, vol. 6, no. 1, 2018, www.corrections.govt.nz/resources/research/journal/volume_6_issue_1_july_2018/where_new_zealand_stands_internationally_a_comparison_of_offence_profiles_and_recidivism_rates.

140. Johnston, Peter. "Book Review: Gangland by Jared Savage." Practice: The New Zealand Corrections Journal, vol. 8, no. 1, 2021, www.corrections.govt.nz/resources/research/journal/volume_8_issue_1_june_2021/book_review_gangland_by_jared_savage.

141. Department of Corrections. "Methamphetamine Use Disorders Among New Zealand Prisoners." Journal of Corrections Research, vol. 5, no. 2, 2017, pp. 11-20. www.corrections.govt.nz/resources/research/journal/volume_5_issue_2_november_2017/methamphetamine_use_disorders_among_new_zealand_prisoners.

142. "Why New Zealand Has so Many Gang Members." The Economist, 14 Feb. 2018, www.economist.com/the-economist-explains/2018/02/14/why-new-zealand-has-so-many-gang-members.

143.   Boomen, Marcus. "Where New Zealand Stands Internationally: A Comparison of Offence Profiles and Recidivism Rates." Practice: The New Zealand Corrections Journal, vol. 6, no. 1, 2018, www.corrections.govt.nz/resources/research/journal/volume_6_issue_1_july_2018/where_new_zealand_stands_internationally_a_comparison_of_offence_profiles_and_recidivism_rates.

144.   "Hāpaitia Te Oranga Tangata | New Zealand Ministry of Justice." New Zealand Ministry of Justice, 16 July 2021, www.justice.govt.nz/justice-sector-policy/key-initiatives/hapaitia-te-oranga-tangata.

145.   "Māori In Prison: Where's The Transformational Change? | Scoop News." Scoop, 29 Oct. 2020, www.scoop.co.nz/stories/HL2010/S00155/Māori-in-prison-wheres-the-transformational-change.htm.

146.   Smale, Aaron. "Why Are There so Many Māori in New Zealand's Prisons?" Longform | Al Jazeera, 2 June 2016, www.aljazeera.com/features/2016/6/2/why-are-there-so-many-Māori-in-new-zealands-prisons.

147.   "Hāpaitia Te Oranga Tangata | New Zealand Ministry of Justice." New Zealand Ministry of Justice, 16 July 2021, www.justice.govt.nz/justice-sector-policy/key-initiatives/hapaitia-te-oranga-tangata.

148.   Waves of Freedom." Vimeo, uploaded by Dash Media, 19 Dec. 2019, vimeo.com/ondemand/wavesoffreedom/380658552.

149.   Nichols, Wallace J. Blue Mind: The Surprising Science That Shows How Being Near, In, On, or under Water Can Make You Happier, Healthier, More Connected, and Better at What You Do. 115-16. Print.

150.   Fields, Howard. "Howard Fields." Profiles, University of California, San Francisco, profiles.ucsf.edu/howard.fields.

151.   Pretorius, Annericke. "Tai Wātea/Waves of Freedom: An Evaluation of a Surf Therapy Programme for High-Risk Males Residing in New Zealand." Master of Health Science in Psychology, Massey University, New Zealand, 2020.

152.   Pretorius, Annericke. "Tai Wātea/Waves of Freedom: An Evaluation of a Surf Therapy Programme for High-Risk Males Residing in New Zealand." Master of Health Science in Psychology, Massey University, New Zealand, 2020.

CHAPTER 6

153.   Post-traumatic stress disorder (PTSD) overview. (2023, July 20). NHS. Retrieved July 29, 2023, from https://www.nhs.uk/mental-health/conditions/post-traumatic-stress-disorder-ptsd/overview/.

154. Horwitz, Allan V. PTSD: A Short History. Johns Hopkins University Press, 2018. Pp 1.

155. Horwitz, Allan V. PTSD: A Short History. Johns Hopkins University Press, 2018. Pp 4.

156. Horwitz, Allan V. PTSD: A Short History. Johns Hopkins University Press, 2018. Pp 4.

157. Young, Harmy of Illusions, 7.

158. "The Job and the Life Research Report." Police Care UK, www.policecare.org.uk/the-job-and-the-life-research-report/.

159. Tourky, M, et al. "Quick Wins to Long-Term Outcomes. an Evaluation of Surfwell for Promoting the Health and Wellbeing of Police Officers." ORE Home, 31 Mar. 2021, ore.exeter.ac.uk/repository/handle/10871/125398. Pp 12.

160. Tourky, M, et al. "Quick Wins to Long-Term Outcomes. an Evaluation of Surfwell for Promoting the Health and Wellbeing of Police Officers." ORE Home, 31 Mar. 2021, ore.exeter.ac.uk/repository/handle/10871/125398. Pp 12.

161. Tourky, M, et al. "Quick Wins to Long-Term Outcomes. an Evaluation of Surfwell for Promoting the Health and Wellbeing of Police Officers." ORE Home, 31 Mar. 2021, ore.exeter.ac.uk/repository/handle/10871/125398. Pp 12.

162. Tourky, M, et al. "Quick Wins to Long-Term Outcomes. an Evaluation of Surfwell for Promoting the Health and Wellbeing of Police Officers." ORE Home, 31 Mar. 2021, ore.exeter.ac.uk/repository/handle/10871/125398. Pp 12.

163. Tourky, M, et al. "Quick Wins to Long-Term Outcomes. an Evaluation of Surfwell for Promoting the Health and Wellbeing of Police Officers." ORE Home, 31 Mar. 2021, ore.exeter.ac.uk/repository/handle/10871/125398. Pp 12.

164. Tourky, M, et al. "Quick Wins to Long-Term Outcomes. an Evaluation of Surfwell for Promoting the Health and Wellbeing of Police Officers." ORE Home, 31 Mar. 2021, ore.exeter.ac.uk/repository/handle/10871/125398. Pp 12.

165. Tourky, M, et al. "Quick Wins to Long-Term Outcomes. an Evaluation of Surfwell for Promoting the Health and Wellbeing of Police Officers." ORE Home, 31 Mar. 2021, ore.exeter.ac.uk/repository/handle/10871/125398. Pp 12.

166. Tourky, M, et al. "Quick Wins to Long-Term Outcomes. an Evaluation of Surfwell for Promoting the Health and Wellbeing of Police Officers." ORE Home, 31 Mar. 2021, ore.exeter.ac.uk/repository/handle/10871/125398. Pp 12.

167. Tourky, M, et al. "Quick Wins to Long-Term Outcomes. an Evaluation of Surfwell for Promoting the Health and Wellbeing of Police Officers." ORE Home, 31 Mar. 2021, ore.exeter.ac.uk/repository/handle/10871/125398. Pp 12.

168. Tourky, M, et al. "Quick Wins to Long-Term Outcomes. an Evaluation of Surfwell for Promoting the Health and Wellbeing of Police Officers." ORE Home, 31 Mar. 2021, ore.exeter.ac.uk/repository/handle/10871/125398. Pp 12.

169. Tourky, M, et al. "Quick Wins to Long-Term Outcomes. an Evaluation of Surfwell for Promoting the Health and Wellbeing of Police Officers." ORE Home, 31 Mar. 2021, ore.exeter.ac.uk/repository/handle/10871/125398. Pp 14.

170. Tourky, M, et al. "Quick Wins to Long-Term Outcomes. an Evaluation of Surfwell for Promoting the Health and Wellbeing of Police Officers." ORE Home, 31 Mar. 2021, ore.exeter.ac.uk/repository/handle/10871/125398. Pp 14.

171. "The Job and the Life Research Report - Police Care UK." Police Care UK - Rebuilding Lives for a Brighter Future, 13 Oct. 2020, https://www.policecare. uk/the-job-and-the-life-research-report/.

172. Tourky, M, et al. "Quick Wins to Long-Term Outcomes. an Evaluation of Surfwell for Promoting the Health and Wellbeing of Police Officers." ORE Home, 31 Mar. 2021, ore.exeter.ac.uk/repository/handle/10871/125398. Pp 14.

CHAPTER 7

173. Autism Speaks. "What is Autism?" Autism Speaks, www.autismspeaks.org/what-autism/what-autism, accessed July 29, 2023.

174. Autism Speaks. "What is Autism?" Autism Speaks, www.autismspeaks.org/what-autism/what-autism, accessed July 29, 2023.

175. Surfers Healing. History. Surfers Healing, https://www.surfershealing.org/history.

176. Surfers Healing. (n.d.). History. Surfers Healing, https://www.surfershealing. org/history.

177. Paskowitz, Izzy, and Daniel Paisner. Scratching the Horizon; A Surfing Life. St Martin's Griffin, 2013. Pp 239.

178. Paskowitz, Izzy, and Daniel Paisner. Scratching the Horizon; A Surfing Life. St Martin's Griffin, 2013. Pp 240.

179. Paskowitz, Izzy, and Daniel Paisner. Scratching the Horizon; A Surfing Life. St Martin's Griffin, 2013. Pp 240.

180. "Cystic Fibrosis." Centers for Disease Control and Prevention, 9 May 2022, www.cdc.gov/genomics/disease/cystic_fibrosis.htm.

181. Cystic Fibrosis." Centers for Disease Control and Prevention, 9 May 2022, www.cdc.gov/genomics/disease/cystic_fibrosis.htm.

182. Cystic Fibrosis." Centers for Disease Control and Prevention, 9 May 2022, www.cdc.gov/genomics/disease/cystic_fibrosis.htm.

183. "Understanding Changes in Life Expectancy." Cystic Fibrosis Foundation, www.cff.org/managing-cf/understanding-changes-life-expectancy.

184. Loose, Terence. "Interview with James Dunlop." Orange County Register, 6 Sept. 2011, www.ocregister.com/2011/09/06/interview-with-james-dunlop-2/.

185. Elkins, Mark R, et al. "A Controlled Trial of Long-Term Inhaled Hypertonic Saline in Patients with Cystic Fibrosis." The New England Journal of Medicine, pubmed.ncbi.nlm.nih.gov/16421364/.

186. "Ambry Genetics: Why Surfing Helps with Cystic Fibrosis." YouTube, YouTube, 8 May 2015, https://www.youtube.com/watch?v=LhBkHK59Fls&t=97s.

CHAPTER 8

187. Christopher & Dana Reeve Foundation. "Stats About Paralysis." Christopher & Dana Reeve Foundation, www.christopherreeve.org/living-with-paralysis/stats-about-paralysis, accessed July 29, 2023.

188. Christopher & Dana Reeve Foundation. "Stats About Paralysis." Christopher & Dana Reeve Foundation, www.christopherreeve.org/living-with-paralysis/stats-about-paralysis, accessed July 29, 2023.

189. Life Rolls On. Spinal Cord Injury. Life Rolls On, https://liferollson.org/spinal-cord-injury.

190. Christopher & Dana Reeve Foundation. "Costs of Living with Spinal Cord Injury." Christopher & Dana Reeve Foundation, www.christopherreeve.org/living-with-paralysis/costs-and-insurance/costs-of-living-with-spinal-cord-injury, accessed July 29, 2023.

191. National Highway Traffic Safety Administration. "Adapted Vehicles." National Highway Traffic Safety Administration, U.S. Department of Transportation, www.nhtsa.gov/road-safety/adapted-vehicles.

192. Life Rolls On. Spinal Cord Injury. Life Rolls On, https://liferollson.org/spinal-cord-injury.

193. "Ted X Youth Featuring Jesse Billauer." https://www.youtube.com/watch?v=m28yt UW6dlw.

194. "Ted X Youth Featuring Jesse Billauer." https://www.youtube.com/watch?v=m28yt UW6dlw.

195. On, Life Rolls. "Life Rolls on: Inspirational Athlete: Adam Bremen." Vimeo, 29 July 2023, vimeo.com/365314223.

196. On, Life Rolls. "Life Rolls on: Inspirational Athlete: Ty Duckett." Vimeo, 21 July 2023, vimeo.com/365316063.

197. RideaWave.org. from https://rideawave.org/.

CHAPTER 9

198. Australian Institute of Health and Welfare. "Mental Health." Australian Institute of Health and Welfare, www.aihw.gov.au/reports/mental-health-services/mental-health, accessed July 29, 2023.

199. Health Foundation. "Children and Young People's Mental Health." Health Foundation, www.health.org.uk/news-and-comment/charts-and-infographics/children-and-young-people-s-mental-health, accessed July 29, 2023.

200. Health Foundation. "Children and Young People's Mental Health." Health Foundation, www.health.org.uk/news-and-comment/charts-and-infographics/children-and-young-people-s-mental-health, accessed July 29, 2023.

201. Wave Project. (n.d.). About Us. Wave Project, https://www.waveproject.co.uk/about-us/.

202. Wave Project. (n.d.). About Us. Wave Project, https://www.waveproject.co.uk/about-us/.

203. "The Wave Project: Evidencing Surf Therapy for Young People in the UK." Global Journal of Community Psychology Practice, vol. 11, no. 2, Apr. 2020.

204. "The Wave Project: Evidencing Surf Therapy for Young People in the UK." Global Journal of Community Psychology Practice, vol. 11, no. 2, Apr. 2020.

205. Community Practitioner, 2015; 88(1): 26–29.

206. "The Wave Project: Evidencing Surf Therapy for Young People in the UK." Global Journal of Community Psychology Practice, vol. 11, no. 2, Apr. 2020.

207. Wave Project. (2022). Impact Report 2022. Wave Project, https://www.waveproject.co.uk/wp-content/uploads/2022/08/Impact-report-2022.pdf.

208. Wave Project. (2022). Impact Report 2022. Wave Project, https://www.waveproject.co.uk/wp-content/uploads/2022/08/Impact-report-2022.pdf.

209. Wave Project. (2022). Impact Report 2022. Wave Project, https://www.waveproject.co.uk/wp-content/uploads/2022/08/Impact-report-2022.pdf.

210. "National Study of Mental Health and Wellbeing, 2020-21." Australian Bureau of Statistics, www.abs.gov.au/statistics/health/mental-health/national-study-mental-health-and-wellbeing/2020-21.

211. McKinley, M. E., et al. (2021). The Impact of Surf Therapy on Mental Health and Wellbeing: A Systematic Review and Meta-Analysis. Journal of Affective Disorders, 283, 318-328. https://pubmed.ncbi.nlm.nih.gov/37211776/

212. McKinley, M. E., et al. (2021). The Impact of Surf Therapy on Mental Health and Wellbeing: A Systematic Review and Meta-Analysis. Journal of Affective Disorders, 283, 318-328. https://pubmed.ncbi.nlm.nih.gov/37211776/

213. McKinley, M. E., et al. (2021). The Impact of Surf Therapy on Mental Health and Wellbeing: A Systematic Review and Meta-Analysis. Journal of Affective Disorders, 283, 318-328. https://pubmed.ncbi.nlm.nih.gov/37211776/

214. Tracks. (2023, February 22). Read how surfing is being used as a mental health therapy. Tracks, https://tracksmag.com.au/read-how-surfing-is-being-used-as-a-mental-health-therapy.

215. McKinley, M. E., et al. (2021). The Impact of Surf Therapy on Mental Health and Wellbeing: A Systematic Review and Meta-Analysis. Journal of Affective Disorders, 283, 318-328. https://pubmed.ncbi.nlm.nih.gov/37211776/

216. McKinley, M. E., et al. (2021). The Impact of Surf Therapy on Mental Health and Wellbeing: A Systematic Review and Meta-Analysis. Journal of Affective Disorders, 283, 318-328. https://pubmed.ncbi.nlm.nih.gov/37211776/

217. McKinley, M. E., et al. (2021). The Impact of Surf Therapy on Mental Health and Wellbeing: A Systematic Review and Meta-Analysis. Journal of Affective Disorders, 283, 318-328. https://pubmed.ncbi.nlm.nih.gov/37211776/

218. McKinley, M. E., et al. (2021). The Impact of Surf Therapy on Mental Health and Wellbeing: A Systematic Review and Meta-Analysis. Journal of Affective Disorders, 283, 318-328. https://pubmed.ncbi.nlm.nih.gov/37211776/

219. McKinley, M. E., et al. (2021). The Impact of Surf Therapy on Mental Health and Wellbeing: A Systematic Review and Meta-Analysis. Journal of Affective Disorders, 283, 318-328. https://pubmed.ncbi.nlm.nih.gov/37211776/

220. McKinley, M. E., et al. (2021). The Impact of Surf Therapy on Mental Health and Wellbeing: A Systematic Review and Meta-Analysis. Journal of Affective Disorders, 283, 318-328. https://pubmed.ncbi.nlm.nih.gov/37211776/

221. McKinley, M. E., et al. (2021). The Impact of Surf Therapy on Mental Health and Wellbeing: A Systematic Review and Meta-Analysis. Journal of Affective Disorders, 283, 318-328. https://pubmed.ncbi.nlm.nih.gov/37211776/

222. McKinley, M. E., et al. (2021). The Impact of Surf Therapy on Mental Health and Wellbeing: A Systematic Review and Meta-Analysis. Journal of Affective Disorders, 283, 318-328. https://pubmed.ncbi.nlm.nih.gov/37211776/

223. McKinley, M. E., et al. (2021). The Impact of Surf Therapy on Mental Health and Wellbeing: A Systematic Review and Meta-Analysis. Journal of Affective Disorders, 283, 318-328. https://pubmed.ncbi.nlm.nih.gov/37211776/

224. McKinley, M. E., et al. (2021). The Impact of Surf Therapy on Mental Health and Wellbeing: A Systematic Review and Meta-Analysis. Journal of Affective Disorders, 283, 318-328. https://pubmed.ncbi.nlm.nih.gov/37211776/

225. McKinley, M. E., et al. (2021). The Impact of Surf Therapy on Mental Health and Wellbeing: A Systematic Review and Meta-Analysis. Journal of Affective Disorders, 283, 318-328. https://pubmed.ncbi.nlm.nih.gov/37211776/

226. FoundationWOW. (n.d.). Our Vision. FoundationWOW, https://www.foundationwow.org/our-vision/.

227. Csikszentmihalyi, Mihaly. Flow: The Psychology of Optimal Experience. Harper and Row, 2009.

228. Csikszentmihalyi, Mihaly. Flow: The Psychology of Optimal Experience. Harper and Row, 2009.

229. Kotler, Steven. The Art of Impossible: A Peak Performance Primer. Harper Wave, an Imprint of HarperCollinsPublishers, 2023.

230. McKinley, M. E., et al. (2021). The Impact of Surf Therapy on Mental Health and Wellbeing: A Systematic Review and Meta-Analysis. Journal of Affective Disorders, 283, 318-328. https://pubmed.ncbi.nlm.nih.gov/37211776/

CHAPTER 10

231. National Oceanic and Atmospheric Administration. (n.d.). Population. Ocean Service, National Oceanic and Atmospheric Administration, https://oceanservice.noaa.gov/facts/population.html.

232. Fenlon, D. (2022, February 15). UK's first artificial wave pool opens in Bristol. Wired UK, https://www.wired.co.uk/article/uk-surfing-artificial-wave-bristol.

233. Warshaw, Matt. The History of Surfing. Chronicle Books, 2010. Pp 473.

234. Warshaw, Matt. The History of Surfing. Chronicle Books, 2010. Pp 473.

235. Warshaw, Matt. The History of Surfing. Chronicle Books, 2010. Pp 473.

236. The Wave. (2022). Impact Report 2022. The Wave, https://www.thewave.com/wp-content/uploads/2023/04/The-Wave-Impact-Report-2022.pdf.

237. The Wave. (2022). Impact Report 2022. The Wave, https://www.thewave.com/wp-content/uploads/2023/04/The-Wave-Impact-Report-2022.pdf.

238. The Wave. (2022). The Impact Zone 2021. The Wave, https://www.thewave.com/wp-content/uploads/2022/03/The-Impact-Zone.pdf

239. Wavegarden Scotland. (2023, March 8). Wavegarden Scotland rebrands as Lost Shore Surf Resort. Wavepool Mag, https://wavepoolmag.com/wavegarden-scotland-rebrands-as-lost-shore-surf-resort/.

240. McManus, J. (2023, February 25). North Berwick and Andrews surf resort mission coming to fruition. East Lothian Courier, https://www.eastlothiancourier.com/news/23345959.north-berwick-andrews-surf-resort-mission-coming-fruition/.

241. Mackay, D. (2023, February 25). Scottish wave pool makes room for university research on-site. Wavepool Mag, https://wavepoolmag.com/scottish-wave-pool-makes-room-for-university-research-on-site/.

ACKNOWLEDGEMENTS

ෙෙෙ

Telling the story of surf therapy, past to present and future, required tremendous effort—and saying to no to surfing more than I preferred. This would book would not have been possible without the help of many people within the sector.

This starts with Kris Primacio, the CEO of the International Surf Therapy Organization. Without you pioneering the 2019 Surf Therapy Symposium in Los Angeles and inviting me to speak, the idea for this book may not have been sown. Kris, you also helped guide and connect me with many organizations in this book. For that, I am grateful, and ISTO—and the surf therapy sector—is blessed to have you, your kindness and your passion at the helm.

I want to thank Ted Silverberg, who welcomed me into his house on a Sunday afternoon on Hawaii's Big Island, turned on live NFL games to watch in the background, and allowed me to dig through photos and other archives that are dear to him. Thank you for your generosity, Ted.

I want to thank everyone who took time out of their days to speak to me about their surf therapy stories. This includes Kris Primacio, Puakea Nogelmeier, Baumhofer Merritt, Ted Silverberg, Mikke Pierson, Jamie Marshall, Carly Rogers, Betty Michalewicz-Kragh, Kristen

Walter, Stephanie Dasher, Justin Martinez, Payton Carty, Jon Ossie, Tim Conibear, Eddie Donnellan, Tim Gras, Tom Losey, Natalie Small, Yvette Curtis, Easkey Britton, Krista Dixon, Jared Dixon, Annericke Pretorius, Howard Fields, James Mallows, Samuel Davies, Jess Miller, James Dunlop, Lynn Labiak, Jesse Billauer, Danny Cortazzo, Carla Miller, Joe Taylor, Joel Pilgrim, Nick Hounsfeld, and Andy Hadden. What an honor it is to be called a pioneer of something in this world— and so many of you are true surf therapy pioneers.

To the Hatherleigh Press team—Andrew Flach, Ryan Tumambing, Ryan Kennedy—thank you for believing in my vision for this book when it was nothing more than an idea, and thank you for guiding me through this publishing process. I'm grateful for your support and insight.

To my wife Celina, thank you for sacrificing by allowing me to spend the proper amount of time required for this book. Thank you for listening to me talk about it for years—the idea itself, what I discovered in my research, the roadblocks that arised, and everything in between. Without your support, this book would not have happened. You are the best wife and mother I could have ever imagined, and some of my most cherished days are the ones we spend together surfing.

To my beautiful daughter Marley, thank you for allowing me to sit inside my writing-cave and do such a time consuming project. My hope is that one day you will understand how fun surfing can be—and therapeutic as well.

To my parents, Tammy and Steve, and my grandparents, Vera and Bill, thank you for pushing me to be a storyteller and communicator since my earliest days. This book is a product of honoring that skill you promoted to me.

While surf therapy is an evidence-based form of treatment, the ultimate treatment for any and every ailment is healing from God. Thank you Jesus for blessing me with the responsibility of this book, and thank you for all the help—there were many instances where I gained access to people, stories and data that truly seemed out of my ability—to help bring this book to life. In truth, you are the actual author of this book, and I'm thankful you allowed me to be your co-author.

And lastly, to every surf therapy practitioner—thank you for all the work, seen and unseen, that you do day in and day out. My hope is that this book inspires and motivates you to keep what you're doing, so that future generations will understand just how powerful surf therapy truly is.

ABOUT THE AUTHOR

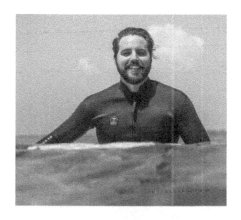

Cash Lambert is the author of Waves *of Healing: How Surfing Changes the Lives of Children with Autism*, published by Hatherleigh Press in partnership with Penguin Random House. He has served in Editorial roles for the last decade. He is the Founder and Director of Editorial for American Surf Magazine. The former editor for Hawaii's Freesurf Magazine, his articles have been featured in ESPN Outdoors, Surfing Magazine, Eastern Surf Magazine, the Outdoor Channel, Surfline, Stab Magazine, Flux, Patagonia and more. A graduate of Palm Beach Atlantic University's School of Communication and Media, he majored in Journalism. Cash lives with his wife, Celina, and daughter, Marley, in Florida.